2·20·79

Surviving Breast Cancer

SURVIVING
Breast
Cancer

Carole Spearin McCauley

 A Sunrise Book · E.P. DUTTON · New York

For information contact:

E.P. Dutton, 2 Park Avenue, New York, N.Y. 10016

Library of Congress Cataloging in Publication Data
McCauley, Carole Spearin.   Surviving breast cancer.
Includes bibliographical references and index.
1. Breast—Cancer.   I. Title.   RC280.B8M25 1979
616.9'94'49   78–15016

ISBN: 0–87690–318–9

Published simultaneously in Canada by
Clarke, Irwin & Company Limited, Toronto and Vancouver

10 9 8 7 6 5 4 3 2 1

First Edition

Contents

2041941

LIST OF FIGURES

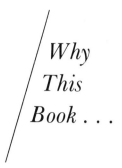

*Why
This
Book . . .*

A major embarrassment of cancer research is its sheer volume.

—P. R. J. BURCH,
professor of medical physics

The most important thing is helping women.

—NATALIA, Chapter 12

As a disease, breast cancer is a welter of paradoxes. It is the leading cause of cancer death among women and the leading cause of all deaths in women aged forty to forty-four—and one of the more curable cancers, *if found early.* Totals have risen to 91,000 new cases—and 34,000 deaths—yearly. Men also get breast cancer.

"We really have made no progress in this disease since 1930 as far as saving lives is concerned," writes Dr. Philip Strax, a specialist in mammography. That is, the percentage of women dying from breast cancer has remained constant for many years (unlike lung cancer, which has increased, and stomach cancer, which has decreased). And the age at which breast cancer strikes seems to be earlier. National Cancer Institute (NCI) data released to author Rose Kushner in 1974 called breast cancer "uncommon under thirty-five, rare under thirty." Now in the late seventies it has become "uncommon under thirty, rare under twenty-five." Indeed, one-third of breast cancer now afflicts women aged thirty-five to fifty. Part of the reason is earlier diagnosis, made possible by the use of mammography.

One of every thirteen American women will get breast cancer, but it does not strike accidentally. Certain women are at higher risk than others, and this book explains the role of factors like diet, hormones, heredity, the age at which a woman first menstruates or bears a child. The book also describes forms of treatment that have proven to be effective alternates to radical mastectomy. One is lumpectomy, followed by various types of radiotherapy and chemotherapy. Another is temporary implantation of radioactive material to destroy malignant tumors. (See Chapter 15.)

This book answers these basic questions:

1. How do you interpret yearly cancer statistics?
2. Is cancer caused by a virus?
3. If caused by environmental pollution, has cancer become epidemic?
4. Which women are at higher risk of breast cancer and why?
5. Is benign breast disease a risk factor?
6. Is cancer emotionally caused?
7. What should you do if you find a lump (new methods of diagnosis)?
8. What alternatives to mastectomy, including non-toxic diet therapies, can you find?
9. Who has organized counseling programs for patients and families?
10. What rehabilitation, including breast reconstruction and physiotherapy following mastectomy, exists?

All this forms, so to speak, the theory behind the book. Its heart, however, is the women themselves. They all were diagnosed as having breast cancer, and received many types of treatment including surgery, irradiation, chemotherapy, emotional counseling, and diet therapy. I also interviewed or learned about women who had rejected orthodox treatment.

Of 3 million Americans alive today following cancer, 2

million have survived five years or longer. Most women in this book are already such survivors. Several praised the honesty and courage of First Ladies Betty Ford and Happy Rocke-feller in admitting their breast cancer. All in this book want to see breast cancer—and mastectomy—out of the closet so women can get effective, humane help *when they need it*—not years afterward. This is the reason they told me their differing stories of medical care and how cancer affected their personal, work, and sexual lives.

Of about 700,000 U.S. women now alive with one or no breasts, one estimate is that only about half—350,000—have come "out of the closet." I offered anonymity, first names, or pseudonyms to all the women I interviewed. Veronica Gardos, for example, wanted me to include her last name. Nearly all chose their own first names. Psychological strength is gained in such honesty, and the women I met spoke frankly with me, knowing their different stories would help others.

Some received excellent care from skillful practi-tioners. All concerned in their cases met the challenge with grace, even occasional humor. Others, however, were out-raged by failures or negligence, among them Natalia, who has sued her physician for $1 million.

Among the women interviewed for this book, I met several whose struggle to obtain compassionate treatment for all cancer patients resulted in action for reforms in care and related issues. Some areas are psychological counseling for pa-tients, monitoring radiation on mammography equipment, two-stage (biopsy separated from mastectomy) operations, an end to radical mastectomy, curbs on environmental pollu-tion, better nutrition, and package inserts to accompany es-trogen drugs.

The spirit and courage these women display while coping with treatment, including physical and psychological recovery from mastectomy, counteract the fear or gloom that surrounds the topic of cancer in many people's minds.

Assembling and blending the raw material of reports, interviews, letters, questionnaires, and data from women who had survived and from physicians, nurses, psychiatrists, social workers, nutritionists, researchers, and librarians on a topic as complicated as breast cancer has been an intense challenge to me. It became an extra challenge because early in the writing, I had to face and negotiate consent forms for both breast and abdominal surgery. Recovery from two surgeons' work consumed more weeks. I was lucky—all tumors and cysts proved benign, as they had previously. I have a history of them.

However, consent forms are structured so that you, while hoping for the best, must assume the worst and either know the terminology or learn it on the spot. Your physician can help—if you meet one willing to explain the range of appropriate treatments. When two-stage operations (biopsy separated from possible mastectomy) or alternate treatments finally become common, women who enter the hospital for a simple biopsy will no longer agonize in the recovery room, wondering, "How much of what did they take off?"

Like other topics of sexual as well as medical interest, breast cancer is a politicized subject with women caught in the middle of the battles over money, research methods, treatments, and aftercare. Radical mastectomy, for example, is not so much a cure as a drastic gamble that excising one-half a woman's upper outline will halt the spread of the disease. Now that alternate effective treatments exist, you deserve to know the facts about them.

The women here show the way . . .

Choose life—
only that and always, at whatever risk.
To let life leak out,
to let it wear away by the mere passage of time,
to withhold giving it and spreading it
is to choose nothing.

—SISTER HELEN KELLEY

KNOWING

1 / *What Causes Breast Cancer?*

In 1977 the number of U.S. women treated for breast cancer as a result of the Breast Cancer Demonstration Detection Projects was revealed. In 280,000 women screened between 1973 and mid-1976, 1,800 breast cancers were found; 592 of these were designated "minimal breast cancer," detected through mammography. And about 60 of the minimal group may have undergone surgery unnecessarily because much minimal breast cancer concerns cells that are in an intermediate phase between being benign and malignant. Some physicians believe such cells are so common that they require no treatment. Dr. Oliver Cope, a surgeon at Massachusetts General Hospital and professor of surgery at Harvard Medical School, wrote:

From a statistical point of view, they can't all be cancers or seeds of real cancers. If they were, cancers of the breast would be much more common, afflicting 20 percent of women instead of 7 percent.

The most frequent tumors of the interphase are minute islands, or clusters of cells too small to be felt or seen by the naked eye. These are sometimes called "multicentric foci," in reference to the several little spots. Under the microscope the cells of these islands are larger than normal cells and look like cancer cells; but they fail to develop into a growing, spreading tumor. They occur in perhaps as many as 30 percent of women at the age of 50. Little is understood of their

3

real nature. I mention them not because I think them dangerous, but
because there is much controversy about them.

The smallest breast lump you or your doctor can feel
is about 1 gram (weight) or 1 centimeter ($^2/_5$ inch), and this
tiny object already contains millions of cells, twenty to thirty
doublings in arithmetic progression from its beginning as one
or more abnormal cells. One estimate by Dr. Ben Byrd, past
president of the American Cancer Society, of the minimum
time needed by a fast-growing breast tumor to reach 1 centimeter is 660 days (about twenty-two months). Abnormal cells
in some breast cancers, however, remain latent for many
years.

Malignant tumors are unpredictable both as to local
growth and their ability to spread. It appears that up to 99
percent of the cells in many tumors may be an inert mass. According to Dr. Sydney Salmon of the University of Arizona
Cancer Center, Tucson:

Not all of the cells in a cancer are malignant and some of the cancer
cells lose their malignant properties of uncontrolled growth and
spread. The key cells of a cancer are called tumor stem cells. The
tumor stem cells can be thought of as the "seeds" of a cancer and
represent the small percentage of total cells in a tumor (often less
than 1 percent) which retain the basic malignant properties. It is the
tumor stem cells that continue to divide and migrate from the primary cancer to other sites in the body and initiate new cancer colo-
nies in a process called metastasis.

Dr. Cope and Dr. Salmon point up the one "fact"
about cancer on which all authorities agree—that knowledge
of the disease is still filled with uncertainties. Before passage
of the National Cancer Act that began the "War on Cancer" in
1971, Dr. Sol Spiegelman of Columbia University confessed in
a hearing before the U.S. Senate: "Our effort to cure cancer
at this time might be likened to trying to land a man on the
moon without knowing Newton's laws of motion. Getting to
the moon was a matter of exploiting existing technology,
whereas curing cancer requires fundamental knowledge we
do not now have."

Contemporary cancer research proliferates with dis-
coveries, facts, and approaches bereft of any acknowledged

unifying theory. Even the statement "Sixty to 90 percent of cancers are environmentally caused" says more about pollution of air, water, or food than it does about the physiology of cancer.

Another way to phrase this: No single theory of hormones, viruses, pollutants, diet, radiation, or genetics presently explains all statistical instances of any cancer, including malignant breast tumors. Factors seem to piggyback upon each other over an individual's lifetime, with some substances as *initiators* and others as *promoters* of cancer. The usual scientific dodge is to call breast cancer, for instance, "multifactorial in etiology" (caused by an interplay of factors). No unifying Einstein of cancer theory has yet appeared.

Agreement is even lacking about whether cancer is one disease or a class of more than 100 diseases. Some crusaders for reform of both cancer treatment and the American diet, like Michio Kushi of the East West Foundation, Boston, believe that what is called "cancer" is not a disease at all. Like fever, it is a symptom of a total disorder that can manifest itself anywhere in the body—chest, skin, breast. During a mumps infection, for instance, the patient runs a general fever but the disease itself settles in, and is fought by, lymph glands in the throat area.

Present biochemical research attacks cancer at three levels: the cellular, the systemic, and the environmental. Yet despite the expenditure of billions of dollars worldwide, the many unknowns about cancer remain unknown. Similarly, the unknowns about breast cancer and its treatment remain the subject of research. Of the ninety NCI-Breast Cancer Task Force contracts funded from November 1976 to November 1977, for instance, at least fifty-four were in experimental biology (study of tumor and normal cell properties, female hormones, etc.) and epidemiology (patterns of incidence, high risk families, possible dietary factors, use of menopausal estrogens, etc.). Additional contracts in these areas were extended without extra funding.

Mary Behr, who has been active in promoting reforms in cancer care (see Chapter 24), points out that "In this country cancer, including related services, has now become a $25-billion-a-year industry. When you consider 1,100 people a day are dying of it, it's apparent we have reached the epidemic stage. But no one seems to be doing much. What a difference when one case of swine flu was detected and twenty-nine people died from 'legionnaires' disease.' Yet most of the money and effort spent on cancer is for treatments *after* we become victims."

This is true if one focuses on research and equipment for surgery, radiation, chemotherapy, even some immunotherapy. Nevertheless, what is primarily wrong with breast cancer research and care is partly what afflicts all U.S. cancer research: lack of humility combined with lack of precise, fundamental knowledge about the biochemical differences between normal and cancerous cells, about body (systemic) changes caused by localized tumors, and about the effects of carcinogens in food, water, air, pesticides, drugs, and other chemicals.

A German surgeon, Auguste Bier, admitted, "There is a tremendous literature on cancer, but what we know for sure about it can be printed on a calling card." Billions of dollars have neither brought nor bought a cancer cure, let alone a preventative. Truth about cancer is unfortunately relative to the beliefs of different people pursuing different lines of research.

Normal Cell into Cancer Cell

The physical process by which one form of virus can turn a normal cell cancerous in just twelve to twenty-four hours was actually photographed in 1976.

This particular "bug," the Rous sarcoma virus that causes a form of cancer in chickens, was discovered in 1910. It possesses one gene that insinuates, or splices, itself into a host cell, beginning the multiple biochemical mistakes that irrevocably alter both the shape and the functioning of the target cell.

Viruses have been called "the ultimately successful cellular guerrillas." In the presence of chick embryo cells and an elevated temperature, Rous sarcoma virus transmuted the observed cells through three stages in photos taken by Eugenia

Wang and Allan R. Goldberg of Rockefeller University, New York. (See Figure 1.)

The first stage began just one hour after temperature rise and lasted two hours. Rufflelike membranes grew and elevated themselves from the region of the cell nucleus. During this stage the chick cells retained their normal elongated (spindle) shape.

Each body cell, human and chick alike, possesses a cell membrane that encloses protoplasm and a nucleus with chromosomes, composed of genes. Genes control physical traits for each species and order the manufacture of enzymes that direct body processes. Each cell is actually a complex chemical factory that uses the foods we eat, plus oxygen, to create amino acids, enzymes, and other proteins. Viruses are genes wrapped in a camouflaging coat of protein.

During the second stage, lasting three to twelve hours, the ruffles regressed or retracted toward the cell nucleus into new structures, called microvilli. These are fiberlike or finger-like projections from the now elevated nuclear region. After more retraction (twelve to twenty-four hours), the spindle-shaped cell became completely round and covered with small blisters, although a few retraction fibers and microvilli remained. At greater magnification of the electron microscope, new viruses and more ruffles appeared to bud from these blisters, ready to attack cells nearby or at distant sites if carried there by the bloodstream.

Such events are both awesome and gruesome. Although no one yet knows the exact mechanism for either fiber formation or change in cell shape, Wang and Goldberg theorize that a gene product called SRC in the virus manufactures a competing protein that attacks the cell's normal muscle protein, ordinarily contained in bundles of elongated structures called microfilaments. Thus its shape is altered until it no longer interacts correctly with nearby cells nor divides normally when the time comes.

This research does *not* mean that viruses cause all or any known specific human cancers or that cancer is contagious like the common cold—only that this particular virus has deformed chick embryo cells and been photographed in

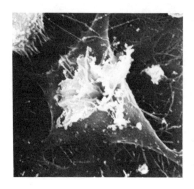 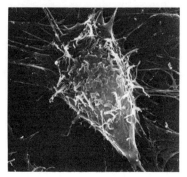

Figure 1. Transformation of a normal cell into a cancer cell in just 24 hours. In the first photograph (above, left), Rous sarcoma virus elevates rufflelike membranes from the cell nucleus one hour after a temperature rise. Photograph 2 (above, right) shows the membranes retracting into fibers, actually changing the cell's shape. In photographs 3 (below, left) and 4 (below, right), at twelve to twenty-four hours, the cell is now completely rounded, with new viruses ready to bud from blisters on the surface and infect other cells. The first three photographs were taken at approximately 1,200-power magnification; the last at approximately 2,400-power. (Scanning electron micrographs courtesy of Dr. Eugenia Wang, Rockefeller University, New York.)

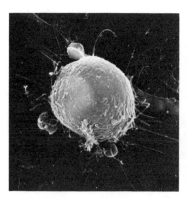 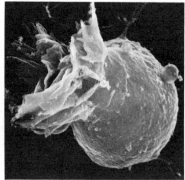

action. However, Dr. Robert Good, director of the Sloan-Kettering Institute for Cancer Research, New York, says: "I don't believe that man is different from the animals. He's just harder to investigate." Photographs also exist of a special kind of white blood cell, the lymphocyte, devouring cancer cells as part of the body's normal immune response. The process, however, is not perfect: some cancer evades detection, and tumors grow.

Despite such research, one of the tragic embarrassments of the much publicized War on Cancer is that scientists do not know—nor can they agree on—the precise biochemical features that differentiate normal human cells from precancerous or cancerous ones.

Some researchers even advise retreat from costly cancer experiments and would replace them with a "back to the biological drawing board" approach. One of these is Dr. Ira Pilgrim, who wrote: "What we know about cancer today is less a function of what the people who have studied cancer have found out than it is a function of what has been discovered about biology in general. The domain of cancer research is, in fact, the domain of experimental biology."

Nonetheless, there are two common characteristics of cancer cells which the photographs of Rous sarcoma virus at work clearly show: derangement of structure and invasiveness of function.

There is nothing pathological about growing a ruffle or even changing cell shape prior to, for example, normal cell division. It is the *purpose* for which the structure or change is intended that determines life or death. Dr. Larison Cudmore, a cell biologist, describes the normal process:

We know what happens when cells touch each other, but we don't know why it happens. In a developing organism, the cells are restless, innately nomadic, and yet extremely polite. If they meet another cell, they stop, refusing to crowd or climb over. To achieve this exquisite courtesy, they have grown a ruffled membrane at their forward end, and this delicate sensor controls the cellular meanderings. If the ruffle touches another cell, its cell is paralyzed motionless until another membrane is grown on another side. It then starts off in that direction, its frilled detector quiveringly sensitive out in front.

Compared with normal cells, malignant ones may have decreased amounts of cytoplasm and bizarre nuclei—larger, doubled, otherwise deformed. Highly malignant tumors have cells with an abnormal number and formation of chromosomes, but these may result from, not cause, the cancerous process.

Cancer cells' deformities as individuals and as a mass make them *less* efficient at life processes, for which they compensate in various ways. One theory holds that cancer doesn't develop in organs where active, normal growth is proceeding but in sites where growth has ceased or lessened, due to aging, as in the breast after menopause.

One path to cancer metastasis is the bloodstream. Tumors are adept at creating their own blood supply. Research of the 1940s reported that

tumor tissue elicited capillary growth as early as three days after implantation, whereas six days elapsed prior to the beginning of capillary proliferation in a wound site.

It is entirely possible that the change in the tumor cell that enables it to evoke capillary proliferation is the only change necessary to give the tumor cell its increased autonomy of growth relative to the normal cell from which it arose.

Here is what happened to a live hamster in research directed by Dr. Solomon Garb, now scientific director, American Cancer Research Center and Hospital, Denver:

The cheek pouch of the hamster, like other mucous membranes, is pink. It has many capillaries. Normally, no large blood vessels can be seen. But after a fragment of cancer had been implanted in our experiments, some remarkable changes occurred. An extensive network of small blood vessels appeared and extended to the cancer. A small artery was apparent within six days, leading from a large artery in the hamster's cheek to the cancer. This newly evident blood vessel began at a site quite distant from the cancer. Within another week, while the cancer grew to the size of a pea, the small artery increased in size until it was as large as the hamster's internal carotid artery, one of the largest in the body.

Indeed, testing whether or not a sample of breast tissue forms new blood vessels when added to host tissue in the test tube may be a way of unblurring the line between benign and malignant cells. In 1977 the National Cancer Institute announced the beginning of clinical trials on this particular "marker for precancerous lesions."

Dr. Mary Sears, an oncologist (cancer specialist) with the Breast Cancer Task Force of NCI, Bethesda, Maryland, has noted that some tumors find body nutrients faster than others and some tumors shed stem cells faster, creating recurrence or metastasis.

How fast is "fast"? One myth about cancer says it is cells run amok, proliferating at rates far beyond normal cells in the afflicted organ. The general rule, however, is that primary tumors arising in a particular organ follow the rate of cell division peculiar to that organ.

For example, healthy red blood cells proliferate rapidly. An average adult has 25 trillion red blood cells, each averaging a life span of 120 days. Over this period, 25 trillion more must be produced to replace aging ones. Mathematically this means the number of red blood cells produced per second in the normal adult is approximately 2,400,000. This amounts to 18 pounds per year. Few tumors attain that weight in twelve months.

Another example of rapid, but benign and orderly, tissue proliferation and differentiation is a seven-pound baby, plus placenta, developing through nine months in the womb. With this in mind, several cancer research projects are studying sperm activity, fertilized egg implantation, and fetal hormone production.

Peggy D. (Chapter 3) is one of the women I interviewed whose history illustrates both the variety of breast cancer and the disagreement between medical pessimists and optimists about how to treat it. After her general practitioner ignored her lump as "nothing serious" for a year and a half, friends and husband convinced her to consult a surgeon. In her own words, by that time, "The tumor was over 5 centimeters [about 2 inches] in size, in fact covered most of the breast. My doctor told me that he was criticized by several colleagues for operating. The usual procedure was [in a tumor of this size] to leave it alone and treat it with drugs. This, I was told, would be an oozing, ulcerated mess by now, if I was still alive.

I am my doctor's 'proof of the pudding.' He had another woman about the same time, who had a very small tumor that ran rampant throughout her body. She is gone. Here I am, still surviving a huge tumor. Cancer has no rules!"

Another tumor characteristic is twisted blood vessels that allow a greater volume of blood within the tumor, compared to normal tissue, but are so structurally irregular that flow is inefficient. This sluggish current in the tumor interior causes the cells there to assume a state similar to hibernation. Indeed, one theory is that such cells—perhaps 99 percent of some tumors—live by fermentation, a chemical process not requiring oxygen at all. If the outer tumor stem cells are killed by chemotherapy or the body's immunological defense system, they are replaced from this inert mass. Following this reasoning, it is easy to see why chemotherapy reaches only some of the tumor cells—those nearest blood vessels or most actively dividing—and is most effective against microscopic tumors.

The Trophoblast Theory

Fetal development has supplied one of the classic directions to cancer research, the trophoblast theory. It was originated by John Beard (1858–1924), a Scottish embryologist, and promoted in the United States by Drs. Ernest Krebs, Sr. and Jr. Briefly, this view holds that cancer is caused not by a virus or other carcinogen but by a normal body cell that begins to act like the *trophoblast.* This is the primitive layer of cells surrounding the fertilized egg that, after its journey down the Fallopian tube, punctures the inside uterine wall and hooks into the maternal blood supply. The trophoblast's second function is to secrete a hormone or other substance which camouflages the embryo and thus prevents the mother's immune system from destroying it for what it is—a partially foreign substance, because it incorporates the father's sperm.

Dr. William Donald Kelley, a nutritionist who recovered from supposedly terminal cancer through diet therapy, is a proponent of the trophoblast theory. He explains why an adult body may still contain these cells.

The placental trophoblast tissue continues to grow until about the seventh week when the baby's pancreas develops. The baby's enzyme production along with the mother's enzyme production stops the growth of placental trophoblast tissue.

As the new embryo is being formed from the normal body or somatic cells, the primitive germ cells are multiplying. In a few days when the embryo develops to the proper stage, the primitive germ cells stop multiplying and begin to migrate to the gonads (ovaries or testes).

There are about three billion of these primitive germ cells that fatigue and never have the vital force necessary to reach the gonads. This means that there are two germ cells for every area the size of a pin head dispersed throughout your body. Any one of these germ cells is a potential cancer. This is why cancer can form in any part of the body.

The trophoblast theory is now discredited because it failed to explain the totality of facts about cancer. Why, for example, do lower animal species like fish, which do not nourish live young through an internal placenta, also get cancer? It has, however, inspired much research in the field of *carcinoembryonic antigens* (CEA). These are substances produced by the surface membranes of cancer cells, including breast cancers. Because the body reacts to them (produces antibodies, as to any foreign substance), researchers hope to use them as markers to betray the presence of a tumor before it can be felt.

The trophoblast theory, then, supposes embryonic cells that escape adult development and reactivate later by themselves perhaps through such carcinogenic stimuli as hormones, improper nutrition, chemicals, or radiation.

Dedifferentiated Cell Theory

The other classic cancer theory, now in favor, involves developed adult cells that revert to an unspecialized, *dedifferentiated* state. All body tissues arise by differentiation and maintain themselves as organs, each performing a specific function (digestion, excretion, secretion of hormones, etc.) under a feedback mechanism of orderly controls. As a result of mutation or other trauma, some cells lose their specialized ability, regress, and form a cancer.

Cells of benign tumors push against other normal cells but do not as a rule push *between* them. (Exceptions to this rule about normal cells are trophoblast cells of the placenta and white blood cells, whose job is migration to sites of injury or infection.) A report on microscopic examination of a benign breast tumor shows what a pathologist looks for:

Sections show portion of mammary tissue with good preservation of lobular architecture [cells as a group have not dedifferentiated]. . . . There is surrounding focal stroma fibrosis [cells in the bed on which tumor rests have encapsulated it with healthy fibrous tissue].

Cancer cells infiltrate and metastasize by somehow modifying the matrix or ground substance in which normal cells lie. They pass between layers of normal cells that are tightly cemented together in this gel-like matrix. They probably accomplish this by secreting, along with toxins (poisons), an enzyme or hormone that eats and digests surrounding cell life.

An example of how this works can be found on your grocer's shelf. Every package of gelatin advises you to avoid fresh pineapple as a fruit filler—to use cooked or canned pineapple only. The biochemical explanation is that fresh pineapple contains an enzyme, bromelin, which destroys gelatin's "gelability."

It is also possible for a tumor that is both noninfiltrating and nonmetastasizing to show the changes characteristic of cancer cells. Judy (Chapter 20) had such a *comedo* carcinoma.

Types of Cancer

Cancer most commonly occurs in body tissues where chemical or reproductive activity is rapid. Such tissues, called the *epithelium,* cover the external body (skin) and internal passages from mouth through intestines. Also included are mucous membranes of the lungs, vagina, and urinary tract, and milk ducts of the breast. Epithelial cells are called *labile* because they normally multiply rapidly to repair wear or damage from passage of food, liquid, and other substances through and past them. Cancer of these epithelial cells is termed *carcinoma.*

In connective tissue, such as bone, cancer is *sarcoma.* In wandering cells like blood or lymph, it is *leukemia.*

It is important to know that breast cancer may be one or even two separate diseases (premenopausal and postmenopausal), further divided into many different kinds of infiltrating tumors. One-half of all breast carcinoma is *scirrhous;* these are the hard, nodule type of cells separated by calcified fibrous tissue. *Medullary* carcinoma is a large, soft tumor composed of cells arranged in glandular formation. It is locally faster-growing but has a better prognosis than scirrhous. *Mucinous* (also called colloid or gelatinous) tumors, filled with a grayish, translucent substance, are the slowest-growing.

Dr. William Sternberg, professor of pathology at Tulane University School of Medicine, New Orleans, has noted, "For a number of years in teaching students, I have illustrated most of the common histologic varieties of breast cancer (scirrhous, medullary, papillary, lobular, mucinous) by showing examples of all these types taken from a single breast." He cautions future doctors on "the danger of basing a prognosis on a single biopsy specimen."

2 / Your Heredity, Hormones, and Reproductive Life

The chemical structure of many of the sex hormones is similar to that of many well-known carcinogenic compounds.

—JOHN WOODBURN,
Cancer: The Search for Its Origins

More and more researchers now doubt that breast cancer originates totally from a single errant cell in a single organ. They are beginning to view it as a systemic disease that focuses on the breast. Many orthodox researchers are approaching the viewpoint, if not yet the practice, of those who uphold alternative or nontoxic therapies such as diet therapy and relaxation exercises to cope with hormone-producing stress. Chapters 2, 4, 6, and 8 focus on what is known of a woman's own "internal weather," as contrasted with larger environmental factors, that may predispose her to breast cancer.

Before consulting the chart of internal risk factors (Figure 2), you should know that:

• The average American woman has a 7 percent (about one in thirteen) *lifetime* chance of contracting breast cancer. (This does not mean that 7 percent of U.S. women get breast cancer yearly. See Chapter 10 for explanations of crude and age-specific rates.)
• By a 1977 American Cancer Society estimate, about

80 percent of women aged thirty to fifty have at least one risk factor. Obviously all these women will *not* get breast cancer. Some combination of factors elevates certain women into the highest risk category.

• The wide range of figures for any factor is due to different results reported by different researchers over the last decade.

Figure 2. RISK FACTORS FOR BREAST CANCER

RISK FACTOR	ESTIMATED INCREASED RISK
Previous breast cancer	3 to 10 times (depending on extent of first disease)
Family history of breast cancer	2.5 to 3 times; 6 to 9 times (if in both breasts or premenopausal in a close relative)
Benign breast disease	2.64 to 4 times
First birth after age 30	3 times (compared to women with first birth before 18)
Early age at puberty (before 11)	2 times
Late age at menopause (beyond 55)	2 times
Childlessness	1.5 times (infertile women)
	1.35 to 2.3 times (single, compared to ever married, women)
Caucasian race, esp. European Jewish or Northern European ancestry	Under investigation
Use of estrogen or progesterone supplements	Under investigation

Previous breast cancer in oneself or close family members (such as mother or a sister) and a history of breast surgery are considered major risk factors. Early puberty, a late first birth, or a late menopause are considered minor risk factors.

Various researchers have linked the following with breast cancer (although no authoritative estimates of increased risk, based on large or wide studies, yet exist): exposure to environmental or therapeutic radiation; urban life; higher socioeconomic status; high fat/protein diet; above-average height and weight; emotional stress; depressive personality; thyroid deficiency.

Now for some good news. Statistically, you have a *decreased* risk of breast cancer if you have:

- No family or personal history of breast disease
- Marriage and childbirth before age twenty-five
- Late puberty
- Early menopause, natural or surgical
- Oriental (Japanese, Chinese, American Indian) ancestry
- A vegetarian diet (although this factor is under investigation).

Much of the available material on risk factors is such a ferment of contradictions that a general guide to major research areas or theories is probably more helpful. One chart I discovered listed "female sex" as the number-one risk factor!

Heredity and Breast Cancer

Ninety percent of breast cancer patients do *not* have mothers or other close relatives (maternal or paternal) with the disease. However, for certain families where the disease strikes several female members and the disease occurs earlier or in both breasts, questions about heredity become inevitable. One woman I interviewed, Mary (see Chapter 22), now in her eighties, had a daughter who also developed a malignant breast tumor.

The first organized research into hereditary factors began in 1866 when a French surgeon, Paul Broca, traced ten of twenty-four women in his family who had died of breast cancer. Seventy years later, the classic study appeared. In 1936, Drs. I. J. Hauser and C. V. Weller published the results of Dr. A. S. Warthin's study of six generations of Family G, whom he termed a "cancer fraternity." In 1936 the family totaled 305 living members, of whom 174 had reached the age of twenty-five—this family's "cancer onset" age. Forty-one individuals (23.6 percent) over that age then had various cancers, including breast cancer. This was a high percentage, especially at a time when breast cancer either was rare or remained undiagnosed, due to ignorance or modesty. However, 25 percent (one in four people) is the current prediction for the percentage of the total U.S. population that will develop some form of cancer. This chilling figure also illustrates why critics of current research rightly believe the disease has reached epidemic proportions.

In 1969, Drs. F. P. Li and J. R. Fraumeni published a study of four families with thirty female members who developed various tumors. Of these, ten were breast cancers. Three mothers in the four families developed this disease before age thirty; of these, two had malignancies in both breasts. (For the range of current age-specific incidence rates, see Figures 7 and 8.)

The single ethnic group most studied for a particular cancer that may be inherited is the Parsi women of Bombay, India; 49 percent of their cancer locates in the breast. Parsi women have also been studied for presence of a viruslike particle in their breast milk that resembles mouse mammary tumor virus (see Chapter 9).

Relatively few U.S. families meet the criteria for high incidence of breast cancer in mother-daughter-sister clusters. By 1976 one researcher, Dr. Henry T. Lynch, had found fifty-two families in which two or more members had breast cancer. These are under intensive study to answer such questions as whether their breast cancers are the same tumor types that afflict the general population; whether they inherit the ability to produce higher levels of certain hormones, particularly estrogens; and whether they produce any substances in their blood or urine (biochemical markers) that could be used to spot early breast cancer in their relatives or other women.

Meanwhile, opinion on genetic links to cancer has not changed substantially in the forty-odd years since Drs. Hauser and Weller's 1936 study, which concluded:

• There are far too many noncancerous children born to cancer patients to support the belief that the cancer trait is determined by inheritance of dominant or recessive genes.

• Nevertheless, there is "strong evidence" that specific body organs may inherit conditions (enzyme or immunological defects, tendency to grow polyps or cysts, hormonal or bone abnormalities) that play host to carcinogens.

In confirmation of this second point, one genetics project at M. D. Anderson Hospital, Houston, Texas, showed that 9 percent of subjects tested had inherited an ability to produce high levels of an enzyme called AHH (aryl hydrocarbon hydroxylase). This enzyme interacts with hydrocarbons in cigarette smoke and converts them to active forms that can induce cancerous growths.

In 1977 another researcher, Dr. John Craig, professor of pharmaceutical chemistry at the University of California Medical Center, San Francisco, reported that "we have recently shown that it is possible to detect, identify, and measure . . . the amount of nicotine and its metabolite found in breast fluid of women within minutes after a single cigarette is smoked." The "breast fluid" need not be milk. It is the normal lymph flowing through the breasts of any woman. A suction pump can obtain a drop of it through the nipple.

I am not stating that smoking causes breast cancer (although it certainly causes lung and throat cancer in susceptible smokers), but because your body functions as a unit, the total effect of any substance like smoke, foods, chemicals, or hormones is cumulative and their interactions are impossible to calculate.

As Dr. Elizabeth Anderson, head of the epidemiology projects section of the Breast Cancer Task Force, NCI, mentioned to me, "The percentage of markers that can be tested for is small, compared to what the body manufactures."

Hormones

Once upon a time, hormones got good press notices, in the days when doctors credited them with responsibility for the longer life span of women compared with men. When further research found a connection between use of the birth control pill and circulatory disorders, benign liver tumors, and breast and uterine cancer in a small percentage of users, women's attitude toward hormones changed.

The most notable breast cancer research projects of the last decade have shown that hormonal interreactions help explain why:

• Women with early menstruation or late menopause get more breast cancer.
• Some Americans and Northern Europeans get breast cancer at rates five times or more that of Japanese and other Oriental women.
• An early first birth protects against breast cancer throughout a woman's life.
• Premenopausal and postmenopausal breast cancer may be two different diseases.
• Some men get breast cancer (about 1 percent of the disease occurs in males).

Nearly a century ago, in 1886, Dr. George Beatson discovered that breast cancer regressed in some women whose ovaries he removed. In younger women, ovaries are the major source of both estrogen and progesterone.

In the 1930s, Dr. A. Lacassagne produced death from breast cancer by injecting estrone (one form or *fraction* of estrogen) into two groups of mice which were unlikely to die of it naturally. One group was male mice. By the 1930s, strains of sister and brother mice, inbred through at least thirty generations and nearly identical genetically, were available to research. Dr. Lacassagne chose two types bred for low (27 percent) and high (72 percent) natural susceptibility to breast cancer. In the highly susceptible strain (cancer would develop in 72 percent of females); he also produced cancer in males with estrone injections that stimulated breast tissue development. One to three months after tumor formation, the male mice died as did the females.

In low-susceptibility females (27 percent develop spontaneous tumors), all the mice died of breast cancer within seventeen months after the estrone injection. In a third series—mice which do not develop breast cancer spontane-ously—none of the animals that survived longer than six months developed breast cancer at all, despite the hormone injections. Some genetic mechanism protected them. Lacas-sagne performed the classic breast cancer research of the thir-ties. John Woodburn, a medical historian, commented:

Lacassagne could not say that large concentrations of estrone caused cancers in all mice. The best he could do was say that, depending on hereditary susceptibility, high concentrations of estrone led to adeno-carcinoma [cancer of glandular cells. By tissue origin, the breast is a modified sweat gland]. Mice highly susceptible because of their ge-netic pattern developed the carcinomas at earlier ages, that is, when lower concentrations of the estrone were present. Animals less sus-ceptible genetically needed higher concentrations of estrone to cause tumors to form.

Researchers have since found that rats are superior to mice for breast cancer experimentation. As in humans, the cancer metastasizes and is more dependent on, or responsive to, natural hormone levels. Rats which become pregnant at an early age are less likely to get breast cancer, even when tumors are induced.

A woman's ages at puberty and menopause are im-portant considerations in estimating her risk of breast cancer. Early puberty (before eleven) and late menopause (after fifty-five) both increase the total time that hormones are active within the body. And the average age of American women at puberty is dropping. Some nutritionists, like Carlton Fred-ericks, believe a girl begins to menstruate when her body reaches a critical weight, which happens sooner today. Ameri-can girls are growing slightly taller with each generation.

Whatever the cause, the average age at first menstrua-tion in the United States has dropped from seventeen about a century ago to twelve and a half years now. And it decreases by two to three months every ten years.

These figures do not include documented cases of precocious puberty occurring in female youngsters aged two to nine. Several of these involved children who regularly swal-lowed their mothers' birth control pills, plus one young lady who at three and a half was using (not eating) "small but regular doses of estrogen-containing face cream." She developed "deeply pigmented nipples and marked bilateral breast development."

The largest study I found that connects age at first menstruation with subsequent breast cancer was done in Caen, France, by Dr. P. Juret and colleagues at the Centre Regional François Bacless (*European Journal of Cancer* 12:9, 9/76). A retrospective study of 926 breast cancer patients between 1958 and 1974, it followed 755 of them for three years after mastectomy. Of these, 647 were traced through five years. Over 100 of the patients were initially excluded from the study because their records failed to indicate their age at puberty. All the women were under seventy at the time of surgery.

Dr. Juret concluded:

Survival rates were the lowest for women who had very early menarche (less than 11 years of age) but prognosis improved progressively with increase in menarchial age. Optimal menarchial age was found to be at age 15; onset of menses beyond this age was once again associated with unfavorable outcome.

A possible reason for this last fact is that abnormally late puberty indicates infertility, hormonal, or nutritional problems.

It is important to understand that estrogen is not the only hormone that affects the breast, especially during the reproductive years. The breast is an organ of both intense and cyclical activity, governed by many hormones, as shown in Figure 3.

The four hormones primarily responsible for breast growth and function are estrogen and progesterone from the ovaries, growth hormone and prolactin from the pituitary.

Estrogen is considered a promoter, rather than an initiator, of breast cancer. If estrogen *alone* caused the disease, no adult female would escape it. A woman who first gives birth after thirty or thirty-five is thought to have an increased breast cancer risk because elevated amounts of estrogen, progesterone, and other hormones needed to maintain pregnancy can affect breast cells already damaged by aging, irradiation, chemicals, and defects in a woman's immunological system.

Biochemically, estrogen divides into three major forms (fractions). Nearly twenty years' research into international differences in breast cancer incidence now points to one of these—estriol—as serving as protection against breast cancer if bound early into breast cells.

How does it get bound?

The answer is one of contemporary endocrinology's detective stories. Among the "detectives" are Drs. Philip Cole and Brian MacMahon of the Department of Epidemiology, Harvard School of Public Health. Dr. Robert Hoover, an NCI epidemiologist who studied at Harvard, told me the story.

Figure 3. BREAST-GOVERNING HORMONES AND
THEIR SOURCES

SOURCE	HORMONE
Ovary	Estrogens, androgens (male hormone)
	Progesterone
Pituitary (base of brain)	Follicle-stimulating hormone (necessary to ovulation)
	Luteinizing hormone (necessary to ovulation)
	Prolactin (milk production)
	Growth hormone
	Corticotropin (acts on adrenal cortex)
	Oxytocin (stimulates birth contractions)
Placenta	Progesterone
	Corionic gonadotropin
	Placental lactogen
Adrenals (atop kidneys)	Cortisol
	Androgens, estrogens
Thyroid	Thyroid
Hypothalamus (forebrain)	Thyrotropin-releasing hormone (acts on thyroid)
	Prolactin-inhibiting hormone
	Gonadotropin-releasing hormone (ovulation)
	Corticotropin-releasing hormone

In the late sixties, after studying both international incidence rates and risk factors for breast cancer, Dr. Mac-Mahon concentrated on data gathered in the early and mid-sixties from areas that are high risk (Boston, Massachusetts, and Wales), intermediate (Greece, Yugoslavia, and São Paulo, Brazil), and low risk (Japan, Taiwan). His initial aim was to see whether breast-feeding protected a woman against breast cancer.

Dr. Hoover commented, "That research destroyed the breast-feeding hypothesis." That is, women who had breast-fed got breast cancer at rates similar to those of their countrywomen who had not. "And it also modified the parity hypothesis," he continued. "Previously it was thought the more kids you had, the more protected you were. Then interest settled on the one statistical fact that did emerge: women who were aged eighteen and under for birth of their first child had one-third the subsequent lifetime risk of breast cancer compared with women over twenty-five at first birth.

"Well, Brian MacMahon presented this information to his classes as a dead end. What did it prove? How did it work? Nobody knew. All MacMahon had done was to destroy both the breast-feeding and the parity myths about protecting a woman from breast cancer.

"Then Phil Cole, an endocrinology student and one of MacMahon's students, came along and assembled the pieces of information into a hypothesis that would explain why an early first birth could be protective."

Cole began with a logical question that would occur to anybody who considers the physiology of pregnancy: How can pregnancy protect against breast cancer *at all* when it increases a woman's estriol production some thousandfold over normal levels?

"As an endocrinologist," Dr. Hoover said, "Phil knew that various kinds of estrogen exist and that they differ in carcinogenic potential. There are twenty-three-plus estrogens but three major fractions—E1 or *estrone,* E2 or *estradiol* [accent on long *i*], and E3 or *estriol* [same long accent]. And estriol, a weak carcinogen compared with estrone, is the major hormone of pregnancy."

Among groups studied (premenopausal and postmenopausal women with and without breast cancer, women at different stages of the menstrual cycle, etc.), Cole and Mac-Mahon compared levels and ratios of the three fractions in women from areas of high breast cancer incidence (United States, Canada, Britain) with lowest risk Japanese and Tai-wanese women. They found a high ratio of protective E3, in comparison to other fractions, in Japanese who remained in Japan. Children of migrants to Hawaii, second or third gener-ation, had intermediate (lower) fractions of E3 and intermedi-ate (higher) breast cancer incidence. Japanese immigrants to the United States had higher rates still.

Was it intermarriage with higher-risk Caucasians, or dietary change to dishes of higher fat and animal protein con-tent that made the difference? If heredity (Mongolian race) were the key against breast cancer, why should it operate in Japan but fail in California? No one blamed U.S. environ-mental pollution, for modern Japan is an urbanized, indus-trialized country. It is also the only country to bear the effects of radiation from two direct atom bomb attacks.

Regarding survivors of the bomb blasts, MacMahon and Cole write:

While it seems clear that ionizing radiation can induce breast cancer in women, the doses have been large in all studies—far greater than those to which most women are exposed—and radiation exposure probably accounts for only a small fraction of human breast cancer cases.

No one knows the answer to this multifaceted puzzle. Herbert Seidman, an epidemiologist at the American Cancer Society, commented to me, "Not only do we lack all the pieces, but the pieces keep changing."

Dr. Hoover says, "It may turn out to be the absolute amount of estrone [the estrogen fraction with the highest car-cinogenic potential] in a woman's system that's important and not the relative amounts of all three estrogens." Thus, a woman who began to menstruate early and experienced menopause late would have five to seven more years of es-trone accumulation.

Drs. Cole and MacMahon's current hypothesis is that

teenage pregnancy binds the good—least carcinogenic—fraction of estrogen early into the breast sites, called receptors, on the surface of cells in a woman's breasts. And it stays bound for life. Pregnancy during the decade after puberty actually makes the breasts biochemically different from those of the woman who gives birth later when her breasts have already bound other estrogen fractions.

This applies to the initial age at giving *birth,* not to pregnancy alone. According to Dr. MacMahon, an abortion before age eighteen seems to increase the risk of later breast cancer.

Compared to research that concentrates on cancer treatment, research into "the hormone connection" gives hope of preventing the disease. While no one can alter the age at which she begins to menstruate, and no adult would advocate increasing the already impressive number of teenage pregnancies in the United States, there is another possibility.

In 1976, Dr. Henry Lemon of the University of Nebraska got approval from the federal Food and Drug Administration (FDA) to locate 10,000 young women willing to try a series of oral doses of estriol to see what effect this would have on future breast cancer rates.

Such work is controversial. Dr. Hoover admitted, "We doctors are good at treating pathology. However, when we try to alter normal physiology, we can screw it up. We just don't know enough about long-term consequences." If the estriol amounts given were less than what a pregnant teenager's body would ordinarily produce or if (Dr. Hoover's suggestion) estriol or estradiol were added to make a safer form of the Pill many young women already use, then risks would be lessened. A new Pill, under animal research since 1972 at the Worcester, Massachusetts, Foundation for Experimental Biology, for example, contains the hormonelike substance prostaglandin instead of estrogen. A woman need take it only once per month instead of daily.

Dr. Hoover stressed the need to integrate all research fields in order to secure some definite answers. "We need a more collaborative effort among biochemists, epidemiologists, endocrinologists, and clinicians. The different fields don't keep up with one another."

Dr. Irwin Vollmer, an endocrinologist and former head of the NCI Breast Cancer Task Force, gave me additional information. "There is tremendous variation in kinds of breast cancer. We may be seeing a new kind now that is environmentally caused, in addition to the breast cancers ordinarily found in women of advancing years.

"We need to check, for example, on all the virus diseases a young girl gets that may act up twenty years later. Generations of women gardeners have been exposed to DDT. It doesn't look like estrogen chemically but it has a slight estrogenic effect. It can promote growth of breast and ovary tissue."

Dr. Vollmer reminded me that only about 50 percent of breast cancers are estrogen-dependent or -receptive, and of those, only 60 percent will go into remission when a woman's ovaries are removed or when she receives a massive estrogen dose that probably blocks prolactin or pituitary hormones feeding her cancer.

Dr. Vollmer noted, "At the dosage at which estriol was found to be noncarcinogenic in mice, it is also noneffective as an estrogen. The amounts given mice should duplicate ratios in the human body. Researchers gave equal amounts of estrone and estradiol, and they should have given higher amounts of estradiol. [Estradiol in the blood plasma of a nonpregnant, fertile woman averages ten times the amount of estriol, for instance.] We need to study the *whole* endocrine system of high-risk women and note imbalances early and not just in the three classic fractions of estrogen. When a woman bears a child, her pituitary hormones are affected, too, not just her estrogen levels."

Researchers who criticize Cole and MacMahon's work point out that estradiol and estrone can easily convert into estriol; that ratios in urinary waste products do not necessarily correlate to ratios circulating in the blood; and that the theory cannot explain the drop in breast cancer incidence after age fifty in Japanese and other Asian populations.

If favorable estrogen ratios were the *main* determinant of a Japanese woman's lowered lifetime risk, then her estriol amount during her teen years should be elevated, compared to a Western woman's. This does not seem to be the case or, more precisely, other researchers do not agree on what it means even if true.

In late 1976, British doctors J. L. Hayward of Guy's Hospital, London, and R. D. Bulbrook, a clinical endocrinologist, published the results of a hormone study in the *European Journal of Cancer* (12:9, 9/76). Dr. Bulbrook had already spent years correlating androgen metabolites in urine samples with subsequent breast cancer in 5,000 women on the Isle of Guernsey, English Channel. He and Dr. Hayward then investigated urine and blood samples from three groups of normal women (no menstrual irregularity, no outside estrogens like the Pill) of three different ages (adolescent, premenopausal, and postmenopausal) in ·Great Britain and Japan.

The results are complex and demonstrate how carefully work must be timed and completed, never forgetting the background question: What *other* factors may be causing or influencing these data?

The difference in the incidence rates of breast cancer in Britain and Japan does not appear to be related to differences in plasma levels of oestrogens or progesterone. . . . The mean excretion of urinary oestrogens in the two races was similar for all groups studied. . . . The only significant difference found in the entire study was that young Japanese girls in the luteal [postovulation] phase of their menstrual cycle had *greater* amounts of oestrone and estradiol in their plasma than did British adolescents. This finding is probably an artefact since the amounts of oestrogen metabolites found in urine collected on the following three days were identical in both groups.

Another researcher, M. B. Lipsett, has suggested that early pregnancy confers its protective "trigger" effect not through a favorable estrogen profile at all but through causing breast cells to differentiate physically via their task of milk production. They remain that way, thereby resisting the dedifferentiation process described in the preceding chapter.

Many researchers feel that it is the total amount of estrogen, rather than certain fractions, that is responsible for increased cancer risk. A woman who receives what gynecologists like to call "an early surgical menopause" (combined hysterectomy and ovariectomy, now done on 25 percent of

U.S. women) has a sharply reduced risk of subsequent breast cancer. According to Dr. Cole, her lifetime risk is decreased 70 percent if the operation is performed before age thirty-five, and 50 percent if done before forty-five.

Some nutritionists believe the dangerous effects of estrogen can be neutralized through diet (Chapter 6), a much less drastic solution than surgery, especially for a young woman who, following a hysterectomy, must take artificial estrogens for the next two decades.

To gain a true picture of a woman's hormonal status, measuring "freed" amounts in the blood or urine is not sufficient. Researchers need some means of measuring how much of which hormones are already bound into body cells. No simple way now exists to gauge the normal (or abnormal) woman's total production or use of hormones over a monthly cycle. One method now in use can test whether breast cancer cells outside the body are estrogen-receptive or not. Another method is radioimmunoassay, which uses a Geiger counter-like machine to follow a hormone given by mouth or injection to see where it goes in the body.

Postmenopausal Breast Cancer

Some researchers consider premenopausal and postmenopausal breast cancer two distinct forms of the same disease or even two different diseases. Postmenopausal breast cancer is related to adrenal misfunctioning, rather than to hormones produced by the ovaries, although a woman's body continues to produce small amounts of estrogen throughout her life.

In 1966, Dr. Charles Huggins of the University of Chicago discovered that premenopausal breast cancer patients whose ovaries were removed continued to menstruate. He found that the adrenal gland produced estrogen in such women and the pituitary had assumed the function of producing prolactin. Other research has suggested that dietary fats are involved in estrogen production for women beyond menopause, since intestinal bacteria can assemble estrogen from steroids in the bile as a by-product of digestive processes (M. J. Hill, "Gut Bacteria and Aetiology of Cancer of the Breast," *Lancet* 1971 II, 472).

Some researchers believe that androstenedione, a hormone from the adrenal cortex, converts to estrone in fatty tissue, and Dr. F. De Waard has postulated that every cell of a postmenopausal woman's body can produce estrogen through metabolizing foods.

A large study of premenopausal and postmenopausal breast cancer is in progress at the University of California at Berkeley, directed by Dr. Ralph S. Paffenbarger. It involves interviewing 2,500 breast cancer patients and 5,000 controls in the San Francisco area with questions about hormone and drug use, family cancer history, age at puberty and childbearing, radiation exposure, body stature, and weight at twenty years of age. But it will be years before the findings are tabulated.

An ingenious piece of research on postmenopausal breast cancer that touches several known factors—hormones, diet, and Oriental women's lowered risk—was done by Dr. John B. Adams of the School of Biochemistry, University of New South Wales, Australia, and published under the title "Steroid Hormones and Human Breast Cancer: An Hypothesis" (*Cancer* 40:1, 325–33, 7/77). Dr. Adams believes that in the development of "Western-environmental" or "adrenal" breast cancer, the crucial hormone is DHEA (dehydroepiandrosterone), secreted and rendered into DHEAS (DHEA-sulphate) by the adrenal gland. This hormone is considered an "estrogen precursor," since mammary tumors can convert it into active androgens and estrogens. Sweat glands in the skin also contain the enzyme needed to metabolize it.

On diet and DHEA, Dr. Adams writes: "In obese subjects urinary DHEA, androsterone, and etiocholanolone [forms of male and adrenal hormone] values are elevated and these values drop upon fasting."

Other work in the late sixties by Dutch researchers A. Hendrikx, W. Heyns, and P. DeMoor demonstrated the effects of a low-calorie diet and fasting upon DHEA in obese women.

The Childless

Statistically, for the premenopausal years, women who have borne children and get breast cancer are more numerous than those who have not. After menopause, however, women who have never borne a child predominate.

Childlessness and breast cancer were first correlated in 1713 by an Italian, Dr. Bernardino Ramazzini. He noted the higher incidence of breast cancer among Italian nuns compared to married women. However, since eighteenth-century nuns did not die in childbirth, as did so many married women, their survival to an older age partially explains their increased rate of the disease.

In 1844, Dr. Domenico Rigoni-Stern of Verona also observed Italian nuns. He wondered whether diet or compression of the breast by clothes or prayer positions upon the stone floors were involved. Because his four male breast-cancer patients were all priests, he suggested a connection between religious orders and cancer incidence.

A nun, Sister Mary Isobel of the Sisters of St. Joseph, Ontario, Canada, who now teaches in a secondary school in northern Tanzania, sent me the following account of her own experience with the disease:

It was early June 1968. The day had been a hectic one at the boarding school where I taught in London, Ontario, followed by a prolonged rehearsal of a play being put on by the young sisters at our mother house.

I was tired, more tired than usual, but then what teacher isn't tired toward the end of the school year? Still, I was exhilarated at the prospect of returning to the University of Notre Dame in Indiana for the summer to complete my M.A. in communication arts.

Suddenly, as I prepared for bed, I became aware that all was not "as usual" with the body I had been carrying about more or less comfortably for 45 years. A strange, tight feeling in one breast, that was all. . . .

After examining her breasts further:

Was it? No, it couldn't be. Besides, it wasn't at all like what I thought it would be. . . . Well, if it was still there in the morning, I would do something about it. But surely. . . .

When the skin tightness remained the next day, she consulted a sister nurse, who referred her to a surgeon, who promised that if he found a simple cyst, she would arrive undelayed at summer school. Unfortunately, the tumor causing the stretched skin proved cancerous. She lost the breast. She concluded:

Well, I didn't get to Notre Dame that summer, but by fall I was able to go back and get that precious M.A. (During the football semester, too—what one of my friends calls a "bonus for good behavior," meaning I suppose Reward for Early Action.)

Sister Mary Isobel was early in finding her disease— and lucky. Because it localized itself to the breast, she needed no postoperative treatment. But as a nun and former cancer patient, she will continue to inhabit the highest risk group of all.

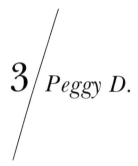

3 / Peggy D.

Like Betty Rollin, author of *First, You Cry,* Peggy D. had a lump which was "watched"—for a year and a half.

By that time, it had enlarged to over two inches and covered most of the breast, inverting the nipple and pulling when she raised her left arm. However, Peggy is alive and well two years following surgery and chemotherapy. Forty-two years old at the time of our interview, she works as a tutor, is married, and cares for a stepson, then age thirteen.

Peggy told me, "After Betty Ford had her mastectomy, I started checking my breasts. I first noticed the lump in August or September of 1974. My general practitioner in Connecticut said it was nothing serious. I had it checked every six months until in November 1975 the nipple began to invert. However, it took until February 1976 for friends and husband to convince me to see another doctor. I went to a surgeon this time."

The surgeon's decision to operate on such an enlarged lump was controversial. "My doctor told me that he was criticized by several colleagues for operating. The usual procedure [in a tumor of this size] was to leave it alone and treat it with drugs. This, I was told, would be an oozing, ulcerated mass by now, if I was still alive." Medical criteria for inoperability were fixed in the 1930s. Major ones include evidence of distant metastasis, inflammatory or ulcerated carcinoma, fixated armpit nodes, positive nodes above the collarbone, or serious prior heart, lung, or kidney disease.

Either because Peggy showed none of these grave signs or because of her youthful age, her new doctor decided on a modified radical mastectomy. "My surgeon and I agreed on this procedure. I didn't want the complete radical, and my doctor didn't want to perform it either." Both frozen and paraffin (permanent) sections of the tumor confirmed its malignancy. (A biopsy of frozen breast tissue usually occurs while a patient is anesthetized. Permanent slides, based on further dissection, are completed a few days later.)

In the hospital, Peggy found the medical personnel sympathetic and generally knowledgeable. "Friends were helpful," she said, "but my parents were shocked. It's difficult for a parent to face the thought (or fact) of their children predeceasing them." However, Peggy's mother rallied, and her assistance improved their relationship. "My mother came to care for me after my return home. I feel closer to her now because of it than I was before."

When I asked Peggy whether she remembered anything particularly comforting or useful someone said or did, she answered, "My husband made a sign with the word PATIENCE on it and made sure it was prominently displayed in my line of vision. I am an impatient person and became discouraged when I wasn't up and going as soon as I wanted to be. Talking to my husband and having his continual support and love was the greatest help."

Knowing she would need further anticancer treatment, Peggy suggested her own after hearing a radio program on new chemotherapy combinations. "I particularly appreciated (and still do) my doctor's openmindedness after I heard on the radio about the CMF treatment [three-drug therapy—cyclophosphamide, methotrexate, 5-fluorouracil—tested postmastectomy in Italy by Dr. Gianni Bonadonna] while I was recovering from surgery. I told him about it. He read up and was willing to try it. I was very ill during my chemotherapy (two weeks on treatment and two weeks off). . . . I got through it all somehow—with a lot of love from family and friends and a *great* deal of prayer."

Peggy continued: "I was lucky in that I returned to

ıy (at that time) part-time job of 1½ hours per day with little difficulty though I was very nervous the first day back. I tried not to take many days off, aware that I felt I had to show the other women that I could be 'normal' and not ill too often. They knew about my situation."

Peggy's present medical care involves a checkup by the doctor every three months ("He checks for lumps, etc.") and a bone scan every six months.

Like others in this book, Peggy fits at least one category of recognized risk factor—no live birth before age thirty. "I have read about this research," she told me. "I have never had a child by birth so I do fit into that category."

Peggy admitted she had "thought about death continuously" during her postoperative and chemotherapy months. Her "turning point" toward life arrived in a way ironically familiar to contemporary Americans: her magazine subscriptions expired, requiring a decision. "I had to face renewing magazines and decided to renew for two years instead of one year only. I made a commitment to survive! Seems trivial, but it was so important to my outlook at that point, perhaps three or four months after surgery. I feel, in part, that *McCall's* and *Ladies' Home Journal* started my mental turnabout toward living beyond just a month at a time."

The grace—and determination—to survive announce themselves in strange ways.

4 / Synthetic Estrogens and Benign Breast Disease

The use of artificial estrogens is a hype to sell pregnant mares' urine at inflated prices.

—BARBARA SEAMAN, radio interview

Kathryn died at twenty-five of metastasized breast cancer. Her mastectomy was so poorly done that her shoulder and chest pain masked the pain of the fatal metastasis.

During her last months of life, she and her mother, Natalie S. Greenfield, prepared a legal suit not against the surgeon but against a drug company that manufactures the Pill Kathryn had taken at her husband's insistence for several months before discovering the breast lump. The suit did not accuse the oral contraceptive of causing the cancer; no one could prove that. Instead, it argued that since Kathryn's tumor was estrogen-dependent, the Pill had speeded its spread.

Kathryn wrote, "If I must die and die so terribly, let me die feeling fulfilled. I want to feel that I've done everything I could to expose the secrecy and silence that exists about the Pill. I want to warn others so they won't be misinformed or suffer the pain and agony I've had."

When the case reached trial, the judge awarded in Kathryn's favor. Her mother donated the money to libraries where Kathryn had researched to prepare her case. Hers was one of the first cases settled in court that correlated Pill usage with some aspect of cancer.

Kathryn did not choose to take the Pill. She agreed to chemical contraception because of her medical student husband's fear of early pregnancy. Had she gotten pregnant, it is likely the hormones of pregnancy would have promoted her tumor just as rapidly as the Pill. However, that speculates on what did not happen and ignores what did. Although her marriage seemed stable, her husband deserted her and left her cancer care to her parents.

Cases like Kathryn's have led Rose Kushner and others to lobby successfully for a package insert that now warns women of the Pill's potential side effects, as cigarette users are warned. Women should know both the contents and the effects of drugs, cosmetics, dyes, and other products they use regularly. Paradoxically this warning leaflet will further protect not consumers, but the drug companies, which can argue that ignorance is no longer an excuse, since everyone who reads is in effect giving informed consent to what she is swallowing.

About 10 million American women take various forms of the Pill. Young women used to receive hormone shots to prevent miscarriage and still receive them to regulate menstruation or to suppress milk production if they do not want to breast-feed. Five million more women take Premarin or other synthetic hormones for menopausal symptoms. These are the commonest forms of *exogenous* (external) estrogens given to women. The research consensus is that these substances operate like their *endogenous* (natural) counterparts: if connected with cancer, they promote the growth of tumors rather than cause them. "They're the fertilizer, not the seed," remarked one doctor.

Epidemiologic studies, both retrospective and prospective, are available from seven different sources in the United States and Great Britain. None of these has found an increase in either benign or malignant breast diseases since widespread use of the Pill and synthetic hormones began. In fact, all except two studies have demonstrated a *decrease* in benign breast disease in women using hormones for two or more years. The overall frequency of carcinoma has been virtually the same as in those groups not taking hormones, with the possible exception of one special subgroup. In one study, women with previous surgery for benign breast disease (a factor that may increase the risk for subsequent cancer) had an increased risk for cancer after six or more years of hormone usage. This finding remains to be corroborated by data from other sources.

In *The Nature of Cancer,* P. M. Sutton, a British researcher, reported the longest controlled animal study I found—rhesus monkeys of both sexes given large estrogen doses for eight years.

This is the largest total dose of estrogens ever administered to living animals. The effect on the breast was to cause very active growth of the cells but even at the end of the experiment there were no tumors at all and no microscopical evidence that any change toward cancer was present.

Dr. Hugh Davis, professor of gynecology and obstetrics at Johns Hopkins, expressed an opposite conclusion: "Breast cancers have been induced on at least five different species of animals by treatment with the same synthetic hormones being marketed in the oral contraceptives."

The Pill has been called "the single most-studied medication in the world" (although controlled tests on Laetrile may someday exceed it). And it has obeyed the pattern associated with new drugs: proven effectiveness in early clinical trials, followed after years of marketing by safety questions concerning long-term use.

In 1977 a British study of 46,000 women (23,000 users and 23,000 controls, begun in 1968) linked the Pill to increased circulatory disorders and death when used by older, but premenopausal, women (*Lancet,* 10/8/77). One conclusion was, "Women who used the Pill continuously for five years or longer had a death rate nearly ten times higher than nonusers and more than three and a half times higher than women who were on the Pill for less than five years."

However, there was *no* increased rate of breast or ovarian cancer in these women.

The Royal College of Obstetricians and Gynecologists
:

• No change in Pill use by women under thirty
• No change in use by women thirty to thirty-five unless they have used the Pill five years or longer and they smoke cigarettes
• Reconsideration of Pill use in all women over thirty-five
• No Pill use for women with a personal or family history of breast or genital cancer.

Some doctors who prescribed oral contraceptives to help manage benign breast disease have retreated from this practice because they now believe either the Pill itself is dangerous to certain women or that benign disease predisposes to malignant. Drs. Elfriede Fasal and Ralph Paffenbarger, Cancer Control, State of California, Berkeley, report in *Journal of the National Cancer Institute* (58:1, 1/77): "Although the experience is limited [a California study of twenty-seven breast cancer patients], it shows that women with a history of prior biopsy for benign breast disease, who had taken oral contraceptives for more than six years, had an elevenfold increased risk of developing breast cancer compared with such women who had never used oral contraceptives." Further evidence correlating synthetic estrogens with cancers of the uterus or breast appeared in *New York State Journal of Medicine* (6/77) *and New England Journal of Medicine* (8/19/76).

Dr. Gary Stein, epidemiology intelligence service officer of the Center for Disease Control, participated in a study in Puerto Rico where Ortho Pharmaceutical plant employees, male and female, were developing high blood levels of estrogen. Five of twenty-five men showed increased levels; three developed enlarged breasts. Of the women, twelve of twenty-three who handled powdered hormone or packed the finished pills experienced unusual vaginal bleeding. Dr. Stein explained, "I doubt very much whether there was any direct ingestion of the substance. But there's a good possibility that skin contact and breathing the airborne particles caused the high estrogen levels in these workers." Whether the exposed workers, both male and female, will show an increased risk for breast cancer, only time will tell.

The Pill remains a safe contraceptive and medication for young women who use it for short intervals. The problem is to spot those who will become high risk for various diseases and equip them with alternate methods of birth control.

Similar advice is now offered for the use of synthetic estrogen during menopause. Despite its longer history of use, the evidence, as with the Pill, remains incomplete because of cancer's even longer latent period in some women. In one study, published in *Today's Health* (5/77), researchers at Harvard, the University of Louisville, and NCI examined the records of 1,891 women seen by one gynecologist over a thirty-year period. Among those who had begun estrogen therapy fifteen or more years earlier, "there were twice as many cases of breast cancer as had been expected." The women in general developed about one-third (30 percent) more breast cancer than expected.

The doctors caution, however, that such data by themselves, without researching other factors, do not indict estrogens as either initiators or promoters of breast cancer but "they raise this risk as a definite possibility." Worded into an FDA directive, the researchers' conclusion is that women with breast or uterine cancer should receive no supplemental estrogen at all, except in special cases where it is used to treat breast malignancy.

I believe there is no point in terrifying millions of women who are already long-term users of the Pill or of menopausal estrogens—and women who will continue to request these drugs from their doctors for immediate health needs. Sensible actions would be to:

- Lower dosages in various forms of the Pill.
- Publicize vitamin substitutes to help menopausal women.
- See that women renewing hormone prescriptions receive regular checkups.
- Urge high-risk women particularly to reconsider prolonged use of any estrogen or progesterone supplement.

Male Breast Cancer

About 700 U.S. men develop breast cancer yearly, and 300 die of it. Although the first figure represents less than 1 percent of breast cancer incidence, the fact that it exists at all in men sheds some light on why women develop it.

Who is the typical male patient—remembering that any average is a composite garment that may not fit particular individuals? Such a man is about sixty years old, and waits ten months before seeking treatment. By comparison, the average female patient is fifty-eight years old and delays only two to four months. The man is probably widowed or divorced, has a drinking problem, and may have sustained a breast injury.

Like female victims, he does not get the disease accidentally. In some men, abnormal estrogen metabolism promotes the growth of tumors, although how they start remains unknown.

One group of men with breast cancer also had prostate cancer, for which they received estrogen to block the effects of the male hormone testosterone on their primary tumor. Some female breast cancer patients are given male hormone for its estrogen-blocking effect.

Men with a chromosomal disorder called Klinefelter's syndrome are at high risk. While the normal male has the sex chromosomes XY among the forty-six in each body cell, the man with Klinefelter's syndrome has XXY sex chromosomes—an extra X, female, chromosome—making forty-seven in each cell. Men with this disorder are sixty-six times more likely to get breast cancer than normal men. Not only does their incidence of the disease approach women's, but it can strike earlier and in both breasts, as it does in female hereditary breast cancer.

Transvestites or transsexuals who receive estrogen to promote breast development face an increased risk of breast cancer, but fear of it should not deter validly motivated people from sex-change surgery. As with female use of the Pill, smaller doses of estrogen and careful, long-term follow-up seem necessary.

The reason widowed or divorced men are more prone to breast cancer was determined by research done in 1963 by epidemiologist Abraham Lilienfeld. Divorced or widowed men are more likely to be alcoholics and develop cirrhosis of the liver. A diseased liver cannot effectively break down by-products of cholesterol and hormone metabolism (see Chapter 6 on diet).

Men with a sudden or chronic injury to the skin and chest may get breast cancer. Typical causes are occupational accidents or a lifetime of wearing suspenders over the nipple areas.

The primary treatment for male breast cancer is radical mastectomy. Compared with women, however, the male survival rate tends to be worse. The disease is more likely to be under the nipple, closer to the chest wall—and reported too late.

Two examples illustrate the risk factors in a man's life. Reported in the medical journal *Breast* (3:2, 4/77) are a father and son, both breast cancer victims. The father had his breasts removed in 1948 and 1952. In 1975 the forty-nine-year-old son had radical mastectomy for a 2-centimeter (3/4-inch) tumor. In 1923 one of the father's sisters had partial mastectomy for breast cancer.

A Washington, D.C., writer, David Rothman, was just thirty years old when he had a mastectomy in September 1977. He had consulted his doctor after noticing a stain on his undershirt when he leaned against a chair arm. Because the twenty-six lymph nodes on the affected side all tested negative for cancer, his doctor gave him the same good chance as a woman for surviving five years—about 80 percent.

In the hospital he wrote:

I am typical of many cancer patients—newly concerned with the welfare of my body.

I'll stop eating my chemical feasts, the junky and processed foods that may have made me more susceptible to the disease.

I'll jog.

And I'll swim.

I think about telling the crowd at the pool that the eight-inch scar across part of my chest and left side is from a duel.

Then I chide myself for not being more fashionable and believable. Why not say the scar is the aftermath of a motorcycle spill?

And finally I criticize myself for thinking of an excuse, period. Why any shame?

He added this chilling paragraph, which describes the probable risk factor in his history:

My parents always saw to it that I received the best medical care. They followed experts' advice in the 1940s and had me exposed to heavy X rays to treat an enlarged thymus (a gland in my neck). It is at least slightly possible that the radiation caused my cancer.

Soon after leaving the hospital, he tested his altered self on a girl friend: "She assures me it won't be worrisome."

Neither David Rothman's mother nor his sister has breast cancer.

In 1977, NCI issued an alert to locate an estimated million Americans exposed to radiotherapy from the 1930s to the 1950s for acne, tonsillitis, and sinusitis when, like David Rothman, they were children. Researchers are especially interested in the increased incidence of thyroid tumors, benign and malignant, in this irradiated population.

Physicians do not see many male breast cancer patients. However, the worries of these men—survival, appearance, effect on loved ones—are exactly those of most female patients.

Breast cancer has—or spares—no gender.

Benign Disease

Several hundred thousand U.S. women will have in-hospital biopsies of suspicious breast growths this year. Statistically, eight of ten such lumps prove benign. One common type of solid benign growth is called *fibroadenoma* (tumor with both fibrous and glandular tissue). Many more women will have fluid-filled cysts aspirated (drained by needle) in doctors' offices or clinics. Whether fluid or solid, a benign lump is noninvasive and theoretically can remain for years without troubling breast or woman.

However, two kinds of breast change, caused by fibrocystic disease at the cellular level, are identified as precancerous. These are an abnormal increase in the number of cells lining one or more milk ducts (*duct epithelial hyperplasia*) and the loss or conversion of normal cytoplasm in some cells into a less differentiated form (*apocrine metaplasia*). Both kinds of change result in cells with abnormal shape, nuclei, and functioning, collectively called *atypia*. Because a small percentage of benign tumors do become malignant or exhibit precancerous changes, some physicians insist on surgical (excisional) biopsy of all lumps, including fluid cysts. They answer, "Absolutely not!" to requests for a needle biopsy of solid lumps or the aspiration of others because they consider benign breast disease a risk factor for cancer development.

Others dismiss it as "a wastepaper basket diagnosis" because of the massive proportion of women—50 percent—who develop fibrocystic disease sometime in their lives. When cysts persist, the condition is called *chronic cystic mastitis*. A California woman, whose mother also had this condition, has all palpable lumps aspirated annually by her doctor, who would biopsy any that refused to aspirate.

Besides fat cells and fibrous tissue, the breast is composed of fifteen to twenty lobes (divisions) of glandular tissue that branch into ducts leading toward the nipple. The anatomy compares roughly to the sections of an orange. Since the whole structure is designed to transport fluid, it is not unusual for some fluid to become entrapped in pocketlike cysts.

Instead of assuming that benign changes can cause malignancy, some researchers theorize that a prior biochemical or hormonal disturbance caused both. Dr. Anaxagoras Papaioannou, author of *The Etiology of Human Breast Cancer,* concludes: "Patients with benign breast disease were found to have the same endocrine abnormalities as breast cancer patients. This is not a causal association, however, and it is more likely that the same noxious factors influence both benign and malignant diseases than that the one condition leads to the other."

Minnie Riperton, a West Coast singer, had a mastectomy in 1976 when she was twenty-eight. She returned to performing and recording despite chemotherapy twice a month and muscle weakness. "I had to learn how to move my arm again. It was numb because they had taken out some nerves." She is the mother of two young children. "When we told the kids," she commented, "my son said he hopes he can be a scientist when he grows up so he can make a bionic breast for me."

Minnie Riperton is one of several thousand women in whom benign and malignant disease are combined. Her biopsy was done with local anesthesia because no one expected such a young woman to need further surgery.

She recalled, "Women have lumps in their breasts all the time. A lot of the lumps are just fibrocystic tumors. Part of mine was a fibrocystic tumor but part was cancer. They found out for sure after the first operation. I was awake through it. Man, what a trip that was.

"I was scared to death at first. Very early in the whole thing, before I had any idea how it would turn out, I looked at myself in the mirror and said, 'Minnie, you're the only one who can make this situation better or worse. You're either going to freak out or you're going to enjoy the rest of your life, however long that may be.' After that day I had a grip on things and it wasn't as hard for me to be cool."

Dr. Oliver Cope (Chapter 15) believes widespread fibrocystic disease in contemporary women comes from "long successions of menstrual cycles uninterrupted by pregnancy." He links it with benign tumors of the uterus because the same hormonal processes or irregularities affect both areas, often simultaneously. "Indeed, one of the ways to substantiate the diagnosis of fibrocystic disorder in the breast is to determine whether the uterus is enlarged generally or harbors one or more fibroid tumors. Forty percent of women in their forties have such uterine changes."

Self-examination is frustrating for women with chronically lumpy breasts. And many, myself included, lack fingers skillful or experienced enough to detect any but the largest cysts (½ to 1 inch). In 1977, I detected a string of three cysts to the side of one breast but missed a 1-centimeter solid lump opposite. My doctor detected it in thirty seconds. Finally I felt it—a movable, BB-like thing, quite different from the soft cysts. It proved benign, but before and after the operation I longed for some nonsurgical method to ascertain its contents—and no pressure to sign the mastectomy consent form until I had at least more knowledge. I signed only for the lumpectomy and removal of the cysts. During the same examination, the doctor also found what finally proved to be fibroid tumors on the outside of my uterus, involving a second consent form (hysterectomy, oophorectomy) to negotiate before the double surgery.

Thousands of women do not need general anesthesia or extended use of operating and recovery rooms for what amount to small lumpectomies. In Europe, needle (incisional) biopsies with fine- or wide-bore instruments are available. They are much less common in the United States because biopsy plus immediate mastectomy on the anesthetized patient, if the lump proves cancerous, is traditional and because many doctors believe invading a lump risks spreading possible cancer when blood or lymph meets cells on the withdrawing needle.

The amount of *money* made by American surgeons, anesthesiologists, and hospitals on probably a yearly half-million excisional breast biopsies that might be done as outpatient procedures under local anesthesia has not gone unnoticed by health reformers. In Rose Kushner's words: "My brief twenty-minute biopsy earned the local surgeon who did it $200, not counting another $30 he got for my office visit and his attempt to aspirate the tumor. . . . That adds up to $2,000 for about 200 minutes of work—or $10 per minute."

The Breast Cancer Task Force of the NCI Division of Cancer Biology and Diagnosis, directed by Dr. D. Jane Taylor, has awarded grants to researchers to study the spectrum of breast problems—"the whole natural history of the disease," to quote Dr. Elizabeth Anderson, an epidemiologist.

We are studying the risk factors of four separate groups of women: those whose tumors are highly malignant; those whose tumors appear to be less malignant; those with benign breast disease that usually has a high probability of progressing toward malignancy; and those whose benign breast disease has a low probability for this progression. For instance, in women who are at low risk of breast cancer, we would like to know whether these people really have fewer benign and premalignant lesions or whether their lesions simply do not progress compared to high risk people.

For women with years of benign tumors or high risk of breast cancer for other reasons, some surgeons now perform prophylactic surgery in the form of a *subcutaneous mastectomy.* The breast contents are scooped out, leaving the skin and the nipple. Shape is restored by inserting an envelope, sometimes prefilled, with silicone or saline solution.

One advocate of this controversial procedure is Dr. Vincent R. Pennisi, a surgeon at the University of California Medical School, San Francisco. He defends it with a study of 711 patients begun in January 1975. Of these, 5.5 percent had, besides benign disease, hidden but invasive carcinoma that would have remained undetected till much later. Another 19 percent had either carcinoma *in situ* or precancerous changes. An additional third of the 711 had a family history of breast cancer or fibrocystic disease. Of the last group, he noted, "All of these might well have gone on to develop frank carcinoma if the surgery had not been performed. The 5.5 percent in whom frank but unknown carcinoma was discovered only as a result of subcutaneous mastectomy is strikingly close to the 7 percent incidence of breast cancer in all women."

Two-thirds of the 711 patients were age thirty-six to fifty. In an interview (*Obstetrics-Gynecology Observer,* 7/77), Dr. Pennisi speculated on hormonal causes:

There may be a triggering mechanism unleashed in this age period, possibly an imbalance between the estrogenic fractions estriol, which is anticarcinogenic, and estradiol and estrone, which are presumed to be carcinogenic. The former declines markedly after age 35, leaving estradiol and estrone unchecked. But in the final analysis, we really don't know what mechanism actually pushes the ductal cell from its orderly behavior to the disorderliness of hyperplasia and, finally, to a malignant change.

The process to malignancy is surreptitious and cannot be detected in its preinvasive state except by chance or by aggressive treatment of fibrocystic disease.

I heard of one woman who had such surgery thirty years ago before silicone reconstruction existed. She has lived her adult life with no breast contents inside the remaining skin.

Some doctors will not consider silicone replacement for contents of a cancerous breast removed by subcutaneous mastectomy, or any mastectomy, for that matter. They believe silicone distorts future examination results—it could mask a tumor on the chest wall, for example. One Connecticut woman I interviewed, Doris, who had a very small tumor, considered either a simple mastectomy (breast removed, leaving nodes and muscles) or subcutaneous mastectomy (breast contents), followed by reconstruction. However, when her surgeon warned, "I can't palpate a breast filled with silicone," she chose the larger operation.

For another view on reconstruction, see Chapter 23.

Now that mammography for the thirty-five-to-fifty age group will be given only to those with a family or personal history of breast cancer, a woman with chronic benign disease has lost a tool that might have provided a few more years' peace of mind. Benign disease is another area that awaits the perfection of a reliable, harmless means of detection, such as thermography or sonography (Chapter 13).

Thousands of American women have had an experience similar to that of a San Jose, California, resident named J.J. The mother of seven children, she had become a first-time grandmother the week I met her. She told me, "I found a lump in one breast. It took me three or four days to get up the courage to make an appointment at the medical center to have it checked. I *thought* I was handling it so well, wasn't getting excited or nervous. The day came. When the doctor finished examining me, I said, '*Is* it?' He answered, 'No. It isn't.' Well, I gave such a whoop. I just burst out!" Here she flung out her arms all over again.

"I had to get a prescription filled at the pharmacy. The pharmacist asked me what I wanted. The first thing I blurted out was, 'I don't have cancer!' Imagine!"

I knew what she meant. One survives those days of suspense, irrationality, and terror, but it helps to have a doctor or family, not to mention a pharmacist, who makes allowances for the tears—or the joy.

5 / Rita: Living with the Diagnosis

Unlike several women in this book, Rita had no history of internal breast disease—no benign tumors or cysts—before discovering a lump in 1971. It was a distinct shock, then, when she learned her doctor's decision to book her for surgery in Manhattan away from her suburban home.

When I interviewed her, she was fifty-eight and the mother of four children who ranged in age from thirty-four to eighteen. She also has one grandson.

Rita discovered her own breast problem. Shivering as she left the shower one evening, she hugged herself to get warm. Her fingers sensed a lump in the lower outer quadrant of her right breast.

First she made an appointment with her internist, who had been the family doctor for twenty years. "He's a very devoted man. He'll even come out in the evening to see patients if they need him." When part of the lump aspirated (drained) successfully and the rest seemed movable, her doctor suggested waiting a few weeks. At the time she was taking "a low dose of Premarin" for menopausal symptoms. He immediately replaced the Premarin with vitamin B6.

At the end of six weeks, when the lump remained unchanged, her doctor decided to book her into Memorial Hospital, affiliated with Sloan-Kettering Institute for Cancer Research, Manhattan. Mammography showed nothing. In fact, a radiologist said, "This is a healthy breast." Yet Rit later proved to be a "false negative." When doctors don't agree on diagnosis, a woman's trauma and confusion can be compounded.

Unlike Irene (Chapter 16), who fought to separate biopsy from mastectomy, Rita wanted a one-stage operation, should mastectomy prove necessary. "The tension would have been too much. As it was, within myself I had to fight constantly about going to Memorial. I really faced the possibility of losing a breast only when *both* breasts were shaved before surgery." In certain cases when an area in one breast proves malignant and is removed, the doctor simultaneously makes a vertical incision down the other breast in search of "mirror tumors." Presence of such a mirror tumor was the reason that Happy Rockefeller's second breast was removed so soon after the first. Rita's surgeon estimates that 20 percent of those with malignant tumors have mirror tumors in the other breast.

Rita had gone into anesthesia not knowing whether she would lose a lump or a whole breast. "I first knew I'd lost a breast when I saw the Hemovac drain in place after I regained consciousness. I spent all day in the recovery room. I returned to my own room only when the private nurse appeared."

Rita had a radical mastectomy of the right breast plus exploratory surgery down the left breast. After the three-day lab work that included nodes from the right armpit, her doctor declared, "All clear." In Rita's case he announced the results carefully, understanding her fear of cancer. He continued, "You had a strange mass in the breast but it had no tentacles." Later, of course, he did use the word "cancer."

When I asked whether she had inquired as to the kind of tumor or why the doctor had performed a radical mastectomy instead of modified radical, Rita replied, "I was not ignorant enough to ignore the problem of a lump but not informed enough to ask all the questions I might have. . . . The hospital experience is a blur. I'd be hard put to say I was on drugs, but I must have been. There's so much to cope with." I assured her that such feelings are probably the average woman's situation, especially if this is her first experience with a lump of any kind.

Rita's psychological adjustment showed some features similar to other women's and some that were particular to her own needs and history. When I asked how she coped with her negative feelings, she answered, "My Catholic faith really meant something to me. I care deeply about religion. My faith was never a burden." Then she admitted, "Well, I didn't have a new baby at forty-one because I thought it was the thing to do. . . . Anyway, when the priest asked me, did I want to go to Confession before surgery, I remember saying, 'I'm at peace.' I was glad I was alive, so there were a lot of feelings I simply didn't have. Fear, yes, but I wasn't angry. I never said, 'Why should this happen to me?'

"On the surface I said, 'I'm putting this behind me.' Underneath, I know I expected death. I don't think even the nurses realize most women are living with the diagnosis, adjusting to it, which medical people interpret as vanity over losing the breast."

Compared with more outspoken women, Rita had difficulty sharing her feelings with her family. She sought to protect both herself and them. "I didn't want to upset anybody at home. The family is so distraught. They feel so terrible for you. The priest told me he has more trouble with the families than with the patients.

"It was difficult for my little one. She was eleven and a half then. We used to lie down together and talk, but she wouldn't do it again for a year afterward. It's more of a shock for a daughter than a son. Doctors began to check her breasts earlier than with other girls. They tend to say things like, 'After your mother's experience, let's just play it safe.' You try hard to forget, but doctors say, 'Not with your history.' "

Once home, Rita faced a new problem—hepatitis from a blood transfusion. Her children noticed her yellowish eyes but refused to tell her, suffering their own unrealistic fears of the disease recurring in her face or head.

Rita was more successful in discussing it with her husband. Since he also had an impairment, a limp that after many years had become simply "a physical fact," Rita devised a comparison. "Ordinarily he's squeamish, but when I considered the mastectomy as resembling in some way his lameness, I could make a joke of going home to somebody who couldn't

stand a Band-Aid. As an Irish Catholic, I always got un-
dressed in the closet anyway, so we didn't have too much
readjusting to do there. With my sisters, however, I never appeared in a nightgown after mastectomy although now I can
with the children.

"Today young people are much more open. It must
be harder for them to adjust to mastectomy if they're used to
appearing without clothes. But I've often thought that if I
were only *thin,* I could walk around naked," she joked. "Anyway, I joined Weight Watchers and have lost some weight."

Unlike some other women in this book, Rita repressed
her feelings in deference to what seemed the good of the family. Nevertheless, emotion tends to burst forth somehow if one
simultaneously hides feelings yet is angered when others don't
notice. When a friend remarked in a phone conversation,
"Gee, you don't look like this other woman I know" (who
seemed ravaged after mastectomy), Rita said, "I burst into
tears. Then I called my friend back to apologize."

Many patients who have surgery in sensitive areas
must gear themselves for tactless comments from embarrassed friends. Rita survived it by recalling advice from a
woman who had been on her hospital floor for a second mastectomy: "What you may find very difficult is meeting people
and seeing pity in their eyes. But if *you* put them at ease—the
responsibility falls on you to do it."

I inquired whether Rita knew of any personal or family risk factors for breast cancer. "I'm the youngest of six. I had
no one in the family—no friend either—who ever had this
surgery." Despite Memorial Hospital's thorough question-
naire, Rita had forgotten one part of her own history until
another friend recalled it. She'd had an eczemalike rash on
the breast that later developed a tumor. A doctor treated it
"for a year" with X rays. Women with mastitis following childbirth also used to receive this supposedly therapeutic irradiation.

While, as with David Rothman (Chapter 4), it cannot
be proved that such irradiation for a skin problem caused
Rita's cancer, her friend's memory and question, "Isn't that
the breast you had the trouble with?" would alarm any woman
in this situation. Such liberal use of X rays for supposedly

therapeutic, instead of diagnostic, purposes has now led to lawsuits where the patient claims her illness was iatrogenic (physician-induced).

"The thing that might have been a risk factor I forgot to tell them," Rita mused.

Like several others in this book, Rita believes radical or modified radical mastectomy "gives more peace of mind" than lumpectomy. "There's greater basis for hope that they got it all." She recalled a TV program in which Barbara Walters interviewed groups of women who had had either lumpectomy or a form of radical mastectomy. Rita commented, "All the radical mastectomy patients, who had recovered satisfactorily, said they did not regret submitting to the larger operation if it had to be done at all."

I wondered whether the years of coping with her situation had changed Rita. "You do have a different perspective afterward," she said. "I'm more patient about many things, housework standards, items like unmade beds in children's rooms. Because of surgery I'm very grateful I'm well enough to help care for my grandson. My daughter works full-time now. Sometimes I think I'm waiting to start living. Once my sister said, 'Did it ever occur to you that you are?' "

Rita summarized a feeling that haunts many people, especially those who have recovered from cancer. "When anything unusual happens, an ache or pain, you don't curl up and die but you feel, I can't possibly grow anything that's nonmalignant. You keep on living but you never stop worrying."

Rita now works in a suburban New York hospital with postmastectomy patients as part of the Reach to Recovery program (Chapter 23). She has served as coordinator of Reach to Recovery volunteers for all of Westchester County.

6 / Your Diet and Diet Therapies

"Breast cancer is a nutritional disease."

I heard this from an epidemiologist at the American Cancer Society. I was interviewing him on domestic and international patterns of breast cancer incidence. The words startled me, for they were more definite than anything I had planned to state about connecting breast cancer with diet. And they resemble what nutritional groups on the far left of the medical spectrum have said for years: Cancer occurs when a body, overloaded with toxins by improper diet, metabolism, or elimination, breaks down through cell mutation.

Whatever one thinks of the programs, politics, or personnel of different nutritional reform groups in this country, they do perform an excellent service in reminding orthodox medical people that cancer is a systemic disease as well as a problem of abnormal individual cells. Treating a few billion tumor cells locally by irradiation or surgery may not be sufficient to save the whole body. Larger—but nontoxic— therapies are needed.

Dr. Robert Hoover, an NCI epidemiologist, remarked, "A lot of international variations of breast cancer may be ascribed to dietary factors." He added that if diet does turn out to be of crucial importance, "One of the less invasive ways to alter breast cancer incidence may be to alter diet."

In 1977 he said, "We wish we were heavily into diet

research. We're starting investigation of an area in rural Nebraska with a high rate of colon cancer." This cancer is ordinarily higher in upper-class urban populations. The Nebraska farm region was settled by Moravians with a dietary pattern different from their neighbors'. In particular, for decades they have brewed their own beer. He commented, "If beer turns out to be a risk factor, it'll break my heart!"

Part of a cancer epidemiologist's job is analyzing data from such "hot spots" (areas of high disease incidence). Are there unusual chemicals in the air or water? What are the local population's reproductive history and dietary patterns? Incidence rates of colon and breast cancer in specific populations tend to be similar and may be related.

Some cancers do seem to occur as a result of (or correlate with) long-term habits of work, diet, reproduction, and recreation shared by general or ethnic populations. Two groups under study because their cancer rate differs significantly from that of other Americans are the Seventh Day Adventists and the Mormons. The typical individual of each group does not drink or smoke. In addition, some Seventh Day Adventist communities are vegetarian, although they do consume eggs and milk. According to Dr. Hoover, their breast cancer rate, unlike their other cancer rates, is not much different from that of the rest of the U.S. white population. "If breast cancer is cholesterol-related, then their breast cancer rate would not drop. Studies of cardiovascular disease and diet may correlate with breast cancer rates."

Diet Implicated in Breast Cancer

In *Charak Samhita*, the seven-volume classic work of Indian medicine, the cause of cancer appears as "excess consumption of dairy food." A diet of whole grains and vegetables was recommended to substitute for animal products and fats.

This was written not last week or last year, by some nutrition group, but *4,000 years* ago! Either there is nothing new under the sun or cancer is, as orthodox researchers claim, a complicated disease in which diet provides one more clue to solving the puzzle.

The diets of two groups of women have proved of special interest to researchers. These are Dutch and other Northern European women, who have the world's highest breast cancer rate, and Japanese women, with one of the lowest known rates.

When Japanese women, whose breast cancer incidence is about one-sixth that of U.S. whites, move to this country, their daughters' and granddaughters' incidence of the disease rises and continues to rise. Since, according to some studies, internal estrogen ratios of Japanese women do not differ much from those of British women of similar ages, factors besides heredity or hormones must operate to explain their initial resistance while in Japan and their better cure rate if malignancy occurs. Among the factors that may be responsible are smaller body stature, less breast tissue, more breast-feeding (which usually prevents ovulation), and better virus resistance.

Other researchers have examined the traditional Japanese diet of fish and vegetables, which is perhaps abandoned by Japanese granddaughters in this country as they acclimate to American school lunches, dormitory dinners, and fast foods in general. It is interesting to note that seafood and kelp, common in the traditional Japanese diet, are rich in the trace mineral selenium—one component of an enzyme that oxidizes and detoxifies the by-products of fats taken into the body.

During a radio interview, Dr. Donald R. Germann, author of *The Anti-Cancer Diet,* stated, "We are eating in a way unprecedented in human history. Nobody knows what the results will be." In particular he discussed caloric excess, including the proportion of fat, in the average American diet. "We get 40 percent of our calories from fat. A Japanese gets 10 to 15 percent. An average American takes in 3,200 daily calories; a Japanese, 2,100." The Japanese daily intake of cholesterol, one component of fat, is 300 milligrams, versus 600 milligrams or more for Americans. One egg yolk has 235 milligrams of cholesterol, for example.

Figures 4 and 5 are charts correlating breast cancer with per capita animal and vegetable fat* consumption, based on United Nations data from the 1960s. Charts for the seventies would not differ substantially: Japan, Thailand, Taiwan, low in animal and vegetable fat consumption and low in breast cancer mortality; the Netherlands, high in all three; United States, Switzerland, and Belgium, similar to each other; Spain and Greece, highest in vegetable fat (olive oil), lower in animal fat, and in the lowest third of breast cancer mortality.

Some countries with low rates of breast cancer possibly underreport both incidence and mortality because of family reticence or inadequate data collection. But even if the statistics were 100 percent reliable, the reader should not conclude that a Japanese-type diet alone helps prevent breast cancer—and possibly other cancers. This would ignore the fate of Japanese men. Over 40 percent of cancer in Japan affects the stomach; gastric cancer alone causes half of Japanese male cancer deaths. An excess of salted, pickled, and spicy foods is considered the promoting factor. However, stomach cancer in the United States for both sexes has declined steadily since the 1900s when Americans—ironically—turned from home-produced, -preserved, or -slaughtered foods to commercially canned or bottled products.

Paradoxical information like this—the same diet that supposedly protects Japanese women kills Japanese men—is one reason you should beware of any claim that cancer has one cause, and therefore one remedy. Possibly cancer is a single disease, but it has various—and too many—causes.

One additional complication in breast cancer research is the disease's lengthy latent period. Thus Japan's present low rate indicates not present risk factors but those that prevailed in the thirties or forties. Possibly in thirty years young Japanese women will approach Western rates.

One researcher who has spent nearly half a century

* Dietary fats are of three kinds. *Saturated* fats (include animal products and the vegetable fats coconut and palm oils) raise blood cholesterol. *Monosaturated* fats (olive oil) lower it but less so than *polyunsaturated* products of vegetable origin (safflower, cottonseed, soybean oils).

Figure 4. ANIMAL AND VEGETABLE FAT CONSUMPTION (GRAMS PER DAY) CORRELATED WITH AGE-ADJUSTED BREAST CANCER DEATH RATES (PER 100,000 WOMEN) THROUGHOUT THE WORLD

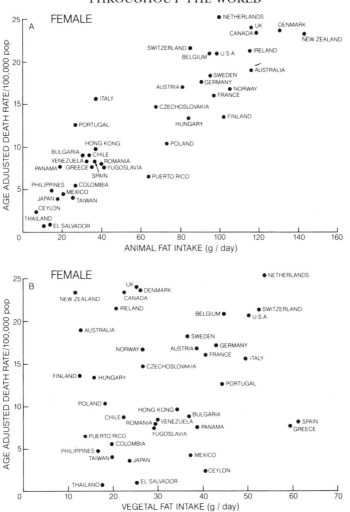

(SOURCE: "Experimental Evidence of Dietary Factors and Hormonal Dependent Cancers," *Cancer Research* 35:3374–83, 11/75 by Dr. Kenneth R. Carroll, Department of Biochemistry, University of Western Ontario, London, Ontario, Canada.)

correlating breast cancer with body weight, stature, and fat intake is Dr. F. de Waard, a Dutch epidemiologist. The Netherlands' mortality rate for female breast cancer is 36.4 per 100,000.*

Figure 5. TOTAL DIETARY FAT CONSUMPTION PER INDIVIDUAL WOMAN CORRELATED WITH AGE-ADJUSTED BREAST CANCER DEATH RATES (PER 100,000 WOMEN) THROUGHOUT THE WORLD

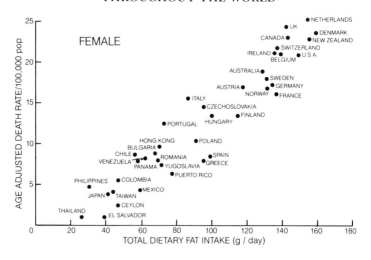

(SOURCE: "Experimental Evidence of Dietary Factors and Hormonal Dependent Cancers," *Cancer Research* 35:3374–83, 11/75 by Dr. Kenneth R. Carroll, Department of Biochemistry, University of Western Ontario, London, Ontario, Canada.)

* U.S. incidence and mortality rates are 74.1 and 29.6 per 100,000, based on 1974–75 data from *World Health Statistics Annual,* 1977, and *Cancer Incidence in Five Continents,* 1976. Average incidence rates are standardized to a European population with a high proportion of older people. The U.S. incidence figure includes tumor registries in Hawaii and Puerto Rico. Within a single country of mixed races like Israel, for example, the female incidence rates for all Jews and non-Jews are 74.2 and 14.6, respectively, again age-standardized to a European population.

Dr. de Waard was the first to publicize one of the mass diet experiments of the twentieth century, which he termed "Adolf Hitler's cancer cure." When the Nazis invaded the Netherlands, they requisitioned most of the cheese, milk, butter, eggs, and meat. The Dutch were forced to live on home-grown vegetables and rationed supplies of staples like white flour, coffee, and sugar.

From 1942 to 1946, Dutch cancer incidence dropped 35 to 60 percent, depending on the district of the country. After the war, as conditions returned to normal, so did cancer rates.

Among the by-products of malnutrition are delayed puberty in girls and the interruption, sometimes cessation, of menstruation in older women. This again illustrates the interrelationship of diet and hormonal levels.

Correlating weight with height, Dr. de Waard has calculated that Dutch women at the top of the scale—the tallest and heaviest, with the greatest body volume—get the most breast cancer. However, no general or simple rule seems to apply. Women 20 or 40 pounds lighter or 6 inches shorter, for instance, do not get breast cancer according to some declining rate based solely on body volume.

Dr. de Waard's work has also correlated the disease with high sugar consumption and related disorders in women aged sixty-five to sixty-nine, and he reports that "in this age group disturbances of carbohydrate mechanism accompanied by obesity and hypertension were found more frequently than in younger women with breast cancer."

Such research may merely confirm cancer's connection with the aging process itself. One theory, developed by biologist Leslie Orgel, holds that aging is the consequence of accumulated errors of information processing in the body. At any point, mistakes can happen at the cellular level. Improperly dividing cells result in "misinformed" genes that order incorrect usage of enzymes or fail to produce those the body needs.

Within the female body, fat deposits contain enzymes that are required to convert androgens to estrogens. (Androgens and estrogens are similar biochemically; it is androgen that creates the normal woman's sex drive.) Dr. de

Waard believes that every cell in the female body, not just fat cells, can produce estrogen. Furthermore, some chemicals and carcinogens are fat-soluble—the body stores them for prolonged periods within fatty tissues.

Bacteria normally present in the intestines can convert various components of bile from the liver into carcinogens. Meat and other heavy foods require longer digestion in the stomach and intestines, therefore more use of bile, than grains and roughage, which transit faster through the body. According to British researcher Dr. Michael Hill, the feces of people on a high fat diet proliferate with certain bacteria which convert cholic (bile) acid into a chemical known to cause cancer in laboratory animals. Dr. Hill estimates that 1,300 grams (nearly 3 pounds) of this chemical would pass through the colon by middle age (fifty years) in a person with a high fat diet.

Some chemicals not known as carcinogenic in themselves may become so when combined with other substances in the digestive tract. A current example is sodium nitrite, added to bacon and other meats to retard spoilage, which forms a compound called nitrosamine. The nutritionist Carlton Fredericks estimates the average American swallows over 5 pounds of food additives (dyes, chemicals, preservatives, etc.) per year. Although small amounts of any one may be safe, no one can calculate the combined effects of all over a lifetime.

Diet Against Breast Cancer

For five years, 100 terminally ill cancer patients at Vale of Leven District General Hospital, Loch Lomondside, Scotland, were treated with large dosages of vitamin C. Dr. Ewan Cameron of that hospital and Dr. Linus Pauling of the Linus Pauling Institute of Science and Medicine, Menlo Park, California, published the results of their research in *Proceedings of the National Academy of Sciences* (10/76).

Each patient began with 10 intravenous grams (10,000 milligrams) of vitamin C daily, then switched after ten days to the same dosage by mouth. The doctors then measured the number of days' survival in these 100 patients, compared to 1,000 controls, matched for factors like age, sex, and kind of tumor, who had not received vitamin C.

The results are startling. Breast cancer patients survived 5.75 times longer, compared with patients in their control group. Instead of averaging only sixty days' life after being declared terminal, these women averaged a year of life. One woman, age fifty, was alive and well four and a half years after starting vitamin C. The control cases similar to hers averaged only eighty-three days.

Drs. Cameron and Pauling wrote: "Our conclusion is that the administration of ascorbic acid in amounts of about 10 grams per day to patients with advanced cancer leads to about a fourfold increase in their life expectancy, in addition to an apparent improvement in the quality of life." And breast cancer patients (along with colon and kidney cancers) even exceeded this fourfold figure.

Vitamin C seems to act by increasing the activity of lymphocytes, which are part of the body's immunodefense system against disease. The vitamin may also strengthen the intracellular cement or gel of normal cells against further invasion by malignancy.

I interviewed one New Jersey woman whose doctor was including large amounts of vitamin C and other nutritional supplements in her postmastectomy recovery program. She stressed the importance of diet for cancer patients to minimize depression, maintain energy, and help their bodies fight the disease. She had returned to work as a college art teacher.

Anticancer dietary programs are usually only one part of a complete health regimen involving preparation of special foods, enemas, and training in relaxation. Two of the best-known programs are taught by Charlotte Gerson Straus, daughter of Max Gerson (*A Cancer Therapy: Results of 50 Cases*) and by Dr. William Donald Kelley (*One Answer to Cancer*). Both recommend use of fresh, raw foods. I met one woman, Carole, who was following this program while negotiating with a surgeon about biopsying a breast lump. Both palpation and mammography had indicated its malignancy. After consulting Mrs. Straus, Carole found a New York nutritionist who recommended a raw foods diet designed to combat cancer and maintain stamina for her life of singing and dance lessons, travel, and irregular hours. She is an opera singer with an established New York company. "At midnight after a performance, I have energy left compared to some others in the cast," she noted.

At a cancer and nutrition conference stressing non-toxic therapies, I also met an ex-breast cancer patient who had been cured four to five years previously after diet therapy, Laetrile, and cellular therapy (a form of immunotherapy), given as injections of serum imported from Germany by her doctor. Another woman named Jessie had been told she had only a year to live, an estimate based on the size, position, and type of her 1-inch tumor. Through a Long Island doctor she began a raw-foods natural hygiene diet that not only checked her cancer but ended some long-term health problems such as monthly breast soreness.

Eydie Mae Hunsberger, a California woman, claims that diet therapy caused her recovery from breast cancer that had visibly metastasized to her underarm. Orthodox medicine tends to dismiss such claims, charging that the patient never had cancer at all or that hers is only one case among thousands and therefore statistically insignificant. Eydie Mae's initial tumor, an irregular lump the size of a quarter under her right nipple, was removed during a biopsy in 1974 when she was in her late forties. The pathology report established its malignancy. Eydie Mae decided against mastectomy—but that is not the point of her story nor of my recounting of it.

Several months later, four new lumps appeared in her right armpit and under the original incision. "The bottom dropped out of my world again," she wrote in an autobiography, *Eydie Mae, How I Conquered Cancer Naturally.* She tried a series of Laetrile injections in Mexico and a combination of immunotherapy, antibiotics, and vitamins. All were ineffective for her. "Pain had now become a daily part of my living."

Through an acquaintance, she learned of Ann Wigmore's Hippocrates Health Institute in Boston, Massachusetts. By law, such an organization cannot and does not practice medicine. It gives nutritional classes, advice, and techniques which students may apply to their own health needs. When Eydie Mae and her husband, Arn, arrived in Boston, she had lost weight, found stairs exhausting, and did not welcome treatment.

Knowing what I do now about Ann Wigmore's program, I don't think I could have gone through it alone and been successful. My energy was at such a low ebb, and my personal discomfort was so great by this time that I really needed the tender loving care and encouragement that Arn provided. Inside me, there was nothing calm, cool, and collected. I was scared and I was desperate.

Lecture classes were attended after breakfast. The classes were usually taught by Ann's paid helpers. We learned a lot about the preparation and combining of raw foods, about enzymes in "live" food (anything raw, seeds, nuts, etc.), how cooking destroys enzymes (important to cancer people because they have a digestive problem especially with protein . . .), how to grow wheatgrass and sprouts, and why we should eat certain foods.

Eydie Mae and her husband learned enough in the days of classes and meal preparation to return to California and begin their own private greenhouse of sprouted wheat and other raw foods. Ann Wigmore bases her therapy on experiments with wheatgrass ingredients, especially chlorophyll and abscisic acid, done by a New Jersey doctor, G. H. Earp-Thomas.

Over a several-month period on the new diet, the cancer cell count in Eydie Mae's urine—one of many tests her doctor performed—steadily decreased. Her weight returned to normal; exhaustion disappeared. By 1975, her tumors had not vanished but had definitely regressed. In 1977, healthy and alive, she was speaking at conferences.

Would Eydie Mae have experienced similar improvement with conventional treatment of mastectomy, chemotherapy, or irradiation? Possibly. Possibly also she is a rare case of spontaneous regression of cancer. Such a miracle occurs only once per estimated 80,000 to 100,000 cases. Two researchers, Drs. Warren H. Cole and Tilden C. Everson, examining thousands of records collected between 1907 and 1962, admitted only 176 (including six breast cancers) to this select group. Spontaneous regression need not imply complete disappearance or cure of cancer, only that the person's body has functioned well over a lengthy period (ten or more years) despite the documented presence of cancer cells. In 1966 the doctors wrote, "Spontaneous regression remains nature's secret."

How does a physician regard a patient like Eydie Mae? Her body's resistance to cancer is attributed to the effective—but unexplained—functioning of her immune system. Here is a typical statement by Dr. James Devitt from a chapter, "Clinical Prediction of Growth Behavior," in *Risk Factors in Breast Cancer:*

The patient who is fortunate enough to have a good tumor-host relationship . . . is less likely to develop local recurrence or distant metastases. If metastases develop, they will occur after a relatively longer "free" interval, and she will survive the metastases for a longer period of time.

Eydie Mae also seems the kind of vigorous, strong-willed personality who would succeed with the psychological approaches against cancer described in Chapter 21.

Another form of nutritional therapy is the macrobiotic diet. Michio Kushi of the East West Foundation, Boston, specializes in cancer treatment through this diet. He writes:

Approximately ten years ago, when I began to study the question of cancer, I investigated the virus theory, the hereditary theory, and various other theories. But gradually I began to realize that none of those analytical, partial approaches could answer the general problem of cancer. . . .

In my opinion, cancer is only the final stage in a sequence of levels of illness through which an individual in the modern world tends to pass because of our failure to appreciate the beneficial nature of disease symptoms. . . . A healthy system can deal with a limited amount of poisonous materials. If, however, we increase the toxins over a long period of time, the body begins to fall back upon more serious measures for elimination: fever, skin disease, and other superficial symptoms. That process of localization is part of our natural healing power, to save us from total breakdown. . . .

It's as if the city-dwellers were to blame the sanitation department for the accumulation of garbage in designated locations, and decided to do away with the sanitation department. . . .

For cancer, as well as other modern degenerative conditions, I would like to suggest the following traditional [Eastern] diet: Every day at least half of our food by volume should be cooked whole cereal grains—brown rice, whole wheat, oatmeal, noodles, etc. Begin the meal with a mildly salty soup containing fermented enzymes: these (traditionally consumed in the Orient in the form of miso, tamari, etc.) help to eliminate toxins. Along with grains we should also, of course, eat vegetables, mostly cooked, but sometimes raw, if desired. As a source of protein, I would recommend beans, and, for minerals, seaweed. Obviously we should eliminate the use of artificially refined products such as white sugar, white flour, and the aptly named "junk" foods. . . . If animal food is desired, it should be limited to small amounts of fish or even poultry rarely—but not red meat.

Michio Kushi has published letters from breast cancer and other patients who have used his program successfully.

Orthodox medicine does not take diet therapies seriously, although the topic of using diet to prevent nausea and weight loss in cancer patients is certainly discussed.

Dr. Stuart Ritchings, a general surgeon on the staff of Kaiser-Permanente, San Rafael, California, who operates daily on cancer patients, had the following to say on nutrition and health food: "Most medical research is for established projects. These often do not include nutrition although intravenous feeding as a nutritional aid for cancer patients is used. Nobody really has hard data on new projects involving vitamin use." He worries about the long-term effects of large dosages of vitamins and admits the conservatism of the medical profession. " 'I think it's a good idea if . . .' is not persuasive without hard data, and even use of this data is conservative."

Ritchings admits that there is a lack of appreciation for preventive medicine in the whole Western medical tradition, although prepaid preventive medical plans, like Kaiser-Permanente in California, are spreading. Unlike doctors in private practice, surgeons in the prepaid system are not paid for increased numbers of operations. Indeed, what they perform must be justified, since the plan must finance every day a patient spends in the hospital.

The Food and Drug Administration regulates about 2,500 additives, 20,000 prescription drugs, 300,000 patent medications, and 4,000 chemicals used in cosmetics. The debate over saccharin use illustrates some roadblocks that afflict food research. Animals, especially laboratory mice and rats, are not people. The amount of carcinogen they must receive to produce tumors in their short life span is massively unlike what a human ingests, and conversely, the range and combination of foods they receive never match human eating patterns.

Carlton Fredericks, a lifetime crusader for improved nutrition, believes that the doctors' tradition of prescribing *single* drugs for ailments, followed by observing specific effects or side effects in a nonlaboratory but nevertheless limited situation, is what hinders their appreciation of a complete dietary program that contains an array of substances. Educated to depend on the healing power of drugs, most doctors are ignorant of the power of foods and supplements. When questioned about nontoxic substances to fight tumors, Dr. James Holland, a New York chemotherapist, replied, "Cancer is an abnormal growth. No normal nutrition can affect it sufficiently. A toxic substance is needed to fight it."

Undoubtedly patients like Eydie Mae, recovered from cancer through diet therapy, use that therapy to continue their favorable tumor-host relationship. Only the most cynical and narrowminded would deny such cures or remissions, even when they come in testimonial form from previously terminal patients. The crucial question is, for how many people does such therapy work—given that some, unlike Eydie Mae, will use it not as an adjunct to surgery but as a substitute for it.

Ruth Sackman of FACT (Foundation for Alternative Cancer Therapies), Manhattan, says, "There are more people in conventional circles doing nutrition work than we realize." This trend will continue as physicians face the limits of conventional therapy and as patients, convinced that some conventional forms of therapy are worse than the illness, demand alternatives.

Nutrition Against Breast Problems?

Whether or not benign breast disease predisposes a woman to breast cancer, there is reason to believe that some dietary substances do prevent breast problems. Dr. Robert London, director of obstetrical and gynecological research, Mt. Sinai Hospital, Baltimore, reported the results of giving vitamin E to a small group of premenopausal women with fibrocystic disease. They received first a placebo, then 600 units daily of vitamin E for two months. Healthy women also received both vitamin E and a placebo (*Obstetrics-Gynecology News,* 12/76). In the fibrocystic women, breast lumpiness decreased during vitamin E use but returned within weeks of stopping the vitamin. Dr. London's explanation is that vitamin E measurably increases the amounts of a hormone secreted by the adrenal gland, and the changed hormonal milieu retards the formation of fluid-filled cysts.

Carlton Fredericks, based on his work with 400 women over twenty years, has developed a complete dietary and nutritional supplement program against breast and uterine problems, which he presents in his book *Breast Cancer: A Nutritional Approach.* His aim is to neutralize the lifetime effects of estrogen in a woman's body: "Instead of removing healthy breasts because they are a target for estrogen, instead of removing ovaries and uteri because they are the producers of estrogen, I advocate placing nutritional brakes on the activity of the hormone."

Fredericks points to excessive estrogen activity as a byproduct of poor nutrition and disturbed liver function. He recommends a diet adequate in protein (including eggs), low in sugar, and high in B vitamins, especially B6. B6 reduces water retention in the breast and helps the liver degrade estrogen and its by-products.

Another recommendation he makes is use of substances like vitamin E, selenium, lecithin, biotin, cholin, and inositol that aid the body in utilizing and excreting fats and in preventing cholesterol buildup. He, too, cautions that "vitamin supplements are not a license for poor nutrition. They are supplements, not substitutes."

One postmastectomy woman remarked to me, "Careful attention to diet not only helps people with cancer feel better. It gives you a sense of recovering your own destiny."

7 / Pat: "You Feel So Vulnerable..."

" 'Pat, you're terrific!' people say to me. Well, what's my choice? I went through this in order to enjoy life by removing as much anxiety as possible." In contrast to other women in this book who were several years beyond mastectomy (although not beyond a fear of cancer recurrence), Pat was just a few weeks beyond her second mastectomy.

Although friendly and willing to be interviewed, she was understandably rushed and tense as she tried to reintegrate all the strands of her life as wife, mother, employee, and ex-patient whose modified radical mastectomy incision was not healing adequately and would probably require plastic surgery.

We began at her Manhattan apartment, then continued the next morning in the coffee shop of the hospital where she is a medical social worker who counsels and assists muscular dystrophy patients with financial and practical life problems.

Pat is one of several women I met who had endured a double—or bilateral—mastectomy. Her first had occurred when she was only twenty-nine, undergoing a divorce, with two small sons, age three and a half and seven, to raise. "When I was told the lump in my breast was cancer, I thought my life as a woman was over. About a year after the operation I met David. A few months later we were married." Indeed, the support of this "special husband" who helped her with necessities like changing dressings was one aspect that made her second mastectomy endurable. The day after that surgery she called me, saying, "The first time I felt like a basket case. This time I'm doing so much better." Pat's two sons are now eighteen and twenty-one. David had three children when Pat and he married.

Her second surgery at age forty-three, fourteen years after the first, qualified as "prophylactic" or "preventive." It was done at her request—not the doctor's urging—when she found a new lump in her remaining left breast. It proved benign but recalled all her terror at the first experience which had begun the same way.

"I'm here now only because of mammography," she emphasized. She discovered the first lump herself while showering. When she saw her gynecologist, he said it was nothing. She objected. "This is crazy. It's something that doesn't belong there. What can we do about it other than surgery?" She knew of mammography and pursued her quest to get the problem noticed, despite a second doctor's declaring he wouldn't even look at the X rays. "If he couldn't feel a lump, that meant it didn't exist. Well, they were right about one thing. That lump was benign."

In the same breast with the benign tumor, however, was a malignant one the size of a pea, and the mammogram showed it clearly to the radiologist. Although routine use of mammography for women as young as Pat with a tendency toward benign tumors (including cysts) remains controversial, in her case it was a life-saving diagnostic tool. She rightly credits it with discovering a malignancy that two different doctors would have ignored until it was much bigger—and much later.

In the present state of the medical arts, patients cannot dictate to physicians which form of diagnosis or treatment they prefer but, armed with knowledge, they can pursue whatever seems intelligent. Too often doctors, including gynecologists who may favor delivering babies over dispensing routine gynecology care, consider women upset about lumps as "crazy ladies." Another reason for this attitude toward breast care is that gynecologists in this country do not ordinarily perform breast surgery; when a lump is detected they are forced to consult or collaborate with a general or specialized surgeon. However, as Patrick McGrady, author of *The Savage Cell,* remarked, "Cynicism has never cured cancer and never will."

Pat continued, "My first concern was living—not the potential loss of a breast." Since no bed was available at a Manhattan hospital that specializes in cancer care, her surgeon booked her into an "acute care hospital" where "they were not prepared for a young woman coming in with breast cancer. The nurses held me at arm's length. My way has always been to get my feelings out. If I felt like crying, I cried. Even my surgeon said, 'You're crying so much you'll get dehydrated.' And I was big on talking about everything."

Pat had a radical mastectomy of the right breast; the nodes in her armpit were healthy and negative for cancer.

She recalled the poor aftercare. "I had nightmares about what to expect under the bandages. They didn't tell me what to expect, about the drains or anything. They didn't tell me to move my arm, so the healing scar tissue formed a web. They didn't recommend any exercise and when I finally did exercise, it was much more painful. They gave me no warning about not allowing vaccinations or injections in that arm so later when we were getting shots for Europe, that arm became an infected mess. . . . Your image has been altered. You feel so vulnerable."

Did anything comforting or useful done for her linger in her mind? She recalled a practical gift from a distant cousin that arrived while she remained hospitalized. It was a handbag. "A noninvalid present for living, a handbag for living in the world again."

I inquired how her friends and relatives had reacted. "I noticed a difference between the women and the men. My male friends or co-workers came to see me first, and they would come alone. The women came later and in a group." We talked about the idea that women feel more threatened than men by another woman's breast cancer and that daughters feel especially threatened. She said, "Yes. Although cancer per se is hard for boys, too. My son, who's eighteen now, let cysts grow on his arm, spine, and back this year without telling me, for instance.

"After my first mastectomy when the children were little, my mother helped a bit. And the neighbors in the suburban place where we lived were helpful. Actually people want to help at a time like that and don't know how. They appreciate clues from the person herself. Speaking my needs if I was feeling blue, not smiling if I didn't feel like it—those things helped me function again. However, I couldn't go and get a prosthesis until I had accepted me and the new image, let's call it. My doctor had to urge me to go and get fitted.

"I was so grateful that mammography and my persistence discovered the tumor early. I felt I'd been given a second chance at living. I left the house in the suburbs and moved with the boys to a small apartment.

"After the mastectomy I began to date men again. And I discovered that after you can tell one person about your experience, you can face it. Yet when it came to the man I loved, I wondered how he would react. But he's a special husband." She smiled. "One year after I was operated on, he fell in love with me."

By the time many women are stricken with breast cancer, one or all of their children are grown and away from home. Pat's boys, however, were youngsters. She commented, "Children have to be told at the level they understand. And they *need* to be told so that they know why you can't pick them up in your arms for a while, so they don't feel rejected or too upset at your moods."

Since Pat's cancer had struck her so young, I naturally wondered what could be known about her personal or family risk factors. The medical facility for Pat's second breast surgery, Memorial Hospital, Manhattan, questions its patients thoroughly on all facets of their histories. "Why, they even ask you whether you had sex before marriage," commented another patient who had breast surgery there (Rita, Chapter 5). One of Pat's aunts had died of breast cancer—in her fifties. Before and after the birth of her sons, Pat had taken "some form of the Pill" for extended intervals. Four years before her second mastectomy, she'd had a hysterectomy to end problems with bleeding and benign fibroid tumors. During the fourteen years between breast surgeries she also suffered from pneumonia and hepatitis.

Whatever role heredity may have played in possibly predisposing her to cancer, Pat seems to be a living refutation of the Cole and MacMahon theory that early pregnancy and childbirth (around age twenty) protect many women from subsequent breast cancer. Whatever protective effect pregnancy in her early twenties conferred seemed to be offset by possible genetic factors or by her "tendency to develop cysts and tumors," both benign and malignant.

Indeed, Pat's history illustrates why all cancer, especially of the breast, is so difficult to research. Although some general risk factors are now known and others suspected, their application to any individual woman's case or course of disease remains speculative, especially over many years' time lapse. Until prospective, instead of retrospective, research can predict or diagnose high-risk women *before* malignant disease develops, those general risk factors which truly apply to the individual woman cannot be known.

During the rest of the interview, Pat and I discussed her second mastectomy experience of a few weeks before. Hot summer weather continued to irritate her underarm incision. "When I found a new lump, in my left breast this time, I consulted both a radiologist and an internist. Mammography indicated it was benign, and my surgeon—the same one I had previously—agreed and wanted only to 'observe it for a while.' He's a wonderful doctor, but the lecture he gave me that amounted to this-breast-is-part-of-your-femininity annoyed me.

"I wanted the same chance I'd had before. I felt if a new malignancy developed, I wouldn't be able to find it in time. . . . If I could make peace with surgery the first time, I guessed I could do it a second time.

"This time my feelings were not shared by other people. My husband and friends tried to dissuade me. People here where I work, however, did understand."

Under pressure, her doctor chose a date for the second mastectomy. As before, her lymph nodes were negative for cancer. In contrast to her previous experience, however,

"I got such devoted care right from the recovery room. I had a private nurse, but by the time she arrived, I was already eating dinner. They encourage everybody to get up, put lipstick on, exercise.

"At first it was a relief to have the ordeal over. Compared with the first time, it seemed like euphoria. But, of course, I came down. When you're tired, you don't have the best handle on your emotions, anyway. I guess I never expected to feel so *vulnerable* all over again." The protracted healing and the possibility of plastic surgery were double factors causing depression. They were preventing her from resuming a full work schedule.

Soon after the surgery, Pat flew to visit her mother in Florida where she recalled some bathing suit adventures. She brought a trio of suits, hoping one or another would work for arm exercise and swimming in a public pool. The zipper of one stuck; her two temporary breast forms popped right out of another in the water. Finally she decided, " 'If people don't want to look at me, they don't have to,' but actually people were understanding. I guess I used to be a more passive person. My present assertiveness has come from all this medical experience."

Again, however, she felt troubled over choosing a permanent prosthesis. "I wanted the smallest possible. I even considered, why bother? Last time I was matching a part that still existed. This time I had nothing to match." I objected, mentioning that without something in the usual places, a woman's clothes don't fall right, that a professional woman like Pat would want to continue to look attractive. She is petite with a wide smile and pixie-cut brunette hair. That day she wore a pastel blue dress with bat-wing sleeves to allow easy shoulder movement.

Feeling it would help other couples, she mentioned one aspect of her marital life. "Naturally I was concerned about sexual relations. I even wanted to keep my nightgown on at first. I said, 'Why remove it?' But my husband reassured me, 'Because it's you. And if you're going to cry, we'll cry together.' " Of the courageous spirits in this book who were able to face the unknown, if not the unbearable, David, whom I met, ranks high.

Besides their own jobs, Pat and David were then volunteering in a couples' counseling group at Memorial Hospital. She also wanted to begin a similar couples' group at her apartment to help others cope with crisis feelings.

We concluded by discussing whether successful confrontation of the problems of the mastectomy period can increase a woman's emotional strength. Pat answered, "Well, I'm certainly more self-assured. I have survived something spiritually—twice now. Each time I had to ask myself what made me a woman before the surgery. And all those qualities are still there."

8 / Psychology and Breast Cancer

Is there a "breast cancer personality"?

Biologists and psychiatrists have debated psychological or emotional theories of cancer causation for decades, if not centuries. Indeed, Galen, the second century A.D. Greek physician-philosopher, was the first to record his opinion that cancer occurred in "melancholic" rather than "sanguine" people. Like so much of cancer research, the materials in this chapter are a focus for continuing debate rather than "received wisdom" agreed on by all.

Cancer is not the only disease for which emotional or stress-related factors are known or suspected. Ulcers, hypertension, and arthritis are other conditions that have been termed *auto-immune,* a way of saying that the body, through some normal process gone awry, begins to attack itself.

In the last few decades, practitioners of psychosomatic medicine have asked whether a recognizable cancer personality exists and if so, whether the personality can be changed before disease develops. Of many researchers, I'll focus on work by Dr. Lawrence LeShan and Dr. George Solomon in the United States and Dr. H. Steven Greer and Dr. G. Nemetti in Europe.

Dr. LeShan's work, reported in his book *You Can Fight for Your Life* and many journal articles, began in the early fifties when he examined personality tests of people who later died of cancer. He noted similarities, particularly in the way patients viewed themselves and their life possibilities. He listed as common factors:

- Loss of a significant central relationship to another person, job, environment, etc.
- Inability to establish new significant relationships
- Inability to express anger or resentment.

He termed this last "immobilization of aggression in one's own defense for one's own needs."

In all the cancer patients seen during the course of my research— over 500—not a single one seemed to have access to more emotional expression than they had energy to express. All seemed to have more emotional energy than they had ways of expressing it. Typically there was a bottled-up quality to their emotional lives. . . .

The emotional force, like an inland pool that has neither fresh inlets nor outward flow, stagnates and becomes a kind of bog in which only organisms of decay can find a home.

By contrast, among LeShan's noncancerous control patients, this emotional pattern was found among only 10 percent.

Included in this life stance are considerable despair and self-pity, summarized by comments like "What I really wanted in life is impossible for me ever to have. What I can have I don't really want. There never really was a way out for me" and "If the rock drops on the egg—poor egg. If the egg drops on the rock—poor egg." Of course, people of all ages occasionally experience such feelings in response to troubles with school, marriage, job, or illness. The dilemma occurs when such an outlook (or inlook) of "quiet desperation" hardens into a permanent life-style.

Dr. H. Steven Greer, senior lecturer in psychological medicine, and Tina Morris of Faith Courtauld Unit for Human Studies in Cancer, King's College Hospital, London, did a study of "Psychological Attributes of Women Who Develop Breast Cancer" (*Journal of Psychosomatic Research* 19:147–53, 1975). A summary of their results reads:

As part of an interdisciplinary study of breast cancer, psychological investigation of 160 women admitted to hospital for breast tumor biopsy was carried out by means of detailed structured interviews and standard tests. . . . Information obtained from patients was verified in almost all cases by separate interviews with husbands or close relatives. Present results are based on statistical comparisons between 69 patients found at operation to have breast cancer and a control group comprising the remaining 91 with benign breast disease. Our principal finding was a significant association between the diagnosis of breast cancer and a behavior pattern, persisting throughout adult life, of abnormal release of emotions. This abnormality was, in most cases, extreme suppression of anger and, in patients over 40, extreme suppression of other feelings. Extreme expression of emotions, though much less common, also occurred in a higher proportion of cancer patients than controls. . . .

These researchers qualified their findings by the following observations:

• Women with benign breast disease may not provide the best control group, since "some social characteristics may be common to women with breast disease per se, whether benign or malignant. Even the assumption that the groups are diagnostically separate is in some doubt, since a small minority of benign breast conditions may be precancerous."

• Extreme expression or suppression of anger may only correlate with, rather than cause, breast cancer. "Statistical associations do not, of course, necessarily imply a causal connection. It must be stressed that no conclusions regarding etiology can be drawn from the preliminary evidence reported here."

• "Previous reports of correlations between breast cancer and extraversion [social conformity], previous stress, and depression were not confirmed."

This final comment connecting breast cancer with variables such as stress, depression, or the use of denial as a coping mechanism refers to research like that done by Drs. G. Nemetti and A. Mezei ("Psychosomatic Studies on Females with Benign and Malignant Tumors of the Breast and Sex Organs," *Psychosomatic Medicine* 5/3–4, 1975). These doctors compared 206 women with cancer of the breast or genital organs with 307 women who had benign tumors.

Characteristics of the cancer group included:

- A greater number of single women
- Unhappy childhoods
- "Only partially satisfactory sex lives"
- Ratings as "good workers" with good relationships to colleagues
- Fewer neurotic or psychosomatic symptoms than the control group.

One conclusion read, "Hysteric conversion reactions, psychopathic behavior, and possible suicide cases were only rarely seen."

The 307 women whose tumors were diagnosed as benign exhibited "more nervousness and other manifestations of hysteria, anxiety, and depression" than did the women with the malignant tumors.

Many psychiatrists, including several I interviewed, do not accept such results or believe them applicable beyond the small groups studied. Much research, especially Dr. LeShan's, cannot answer such questions as, What about people with "cancer personalities" who do not get the disease at all or get something else? and Who can say that fear of biopsy or diagnosis of cancer does not provoke the feelings (panic, depression, anger) then studied?

Cancer patients can be helped to take *responsibility* for emotions in the future course of their illness, as Dr. Simonton explains in Chapter 21. But any diagnosis that merely results in *guilt* for specific past events ("If only I hadn't worried so much when my mother died . . . when I got a divorce . . . ," etc.) seems useless.

A dissenter to the view of cancer as psychosomatic is Dr. Frida G. Surawicz of the Department of Psychology, University of Kentucky College of Medicine, Lexington. Her article "Women, Cancer, and Emotions" appeared in *Journal of the American Medical Women's Association* (32[1]:18, 1/77).

She wrote, "Cancers of the female organs were initially viewed as the somatic expressions of unresolved psychosexual conflicts. The view of cancer as a psychosomatic disease is simplistic as well as speculative and has not been convincingly proven." She also noted, "While the influence of emotional conflict in the development of cancer remains questionable, there is no doubt about the effect of the cancer on the patient's emotional life."

Regarding depression, I find it hard to separate the depression of the cancer patient, who is usually middle-aged, from a common symptom of middle age—the realization that one hasn't, and probably won't, achieve all one desires in job, marriage, or family life.

Regarding overexpression or underexpression of emotion, sexual inhibition, frustration with sex life, etc., these are problems that seem intrinsic to the conventional female roles. Women, as mothers, secretaries, nurses, waitresses, salesclerks, are rewarded for, or at least expected to show, smiling compliance with others' requests and needs. The feminist movement has pointed out the absurdity of the idea that women are supposed to be simultaneously more emotional than men and yet adept at suppressing their own feelings and needs in favor of lifetime catering to husbands, relatives, and bosses.

Cancer and Stress

A wiser approach is to investigate the role of stressful life events in upsetting normal physical or hormonal functioning. Some studies seek to clarify the relationship of stress, depression, and women's status in society—what might be called the *social* psychology of breast cancer.

In *Notes of a Feminist Therapist*, Elizabeth Friar Williams connects hormonal patterns with her patients' feelings of victimization, hopelessness, and loss of self-esteem.

Most psychotherapists agree that women appear more often than men for treatment for depression and more often for depression than for any other psychological problem. . . .

Although it may be true that men's depression often takes physical forms, my view is that women *are* more often depressed than men, for many reasons. For one thing, depression is a condition that is certainly aggravated if not actually engendered by the influence of sex hormones on the pituitary gland, which in turn produces other hormones, particularly norepinephrine, present in the body at high levels in depression. This produces a vicious circle, since depression itself seems to raise levels of norepinephrine and in addition diminishes the body's efficient utilization of vitamins, particularly the B vitamins. . . . This is the reason for the feeling of apathy that most people experience when they are depressed, and it is why they are more susceptible when depressed to the viruses. . . .

Sex hormone influences have been crucially implicated in the notorious depressions of some women at such significant developmental events as menarche, childbirth, and menopause. Currently, however, most people attribute these depressions to women's negative attitudes toward the new roles resulting from these life-style changes. . . .

I disagree. I think psychological attitudes are important at all stages of life, but I believe the chief cause of distress at these significant periods is a change in hormone level and not in sex role. . . . To overemphasize women's feelings about themselves as the source of their troubles is once again to reinforce women's inclination to blame themselves for everything.

Do further biochemical explanations exist?

By popular definition, stress involves a disagreeable event that puts you under tension. By scientific definition, however, stress is a physical response to any kind of demand, pleasant as well as unpleasant. According to Dr. Hans Selye, the stress specialist in Montreal, Canada, complete absence of stress does not and should not exist in life. Even in sleep, functions of respiration, heartbeat, and brain waves continue.

Mere nervous tension or worry is *not* stress unless it produces some body response, such as release of hormones (he calls them *corticoids*) that increase blood pressure and prepare the body for some challenge, fight, flight. Many current biofeedback, meditation, and relaxation techniques operate from the assumption that while you cannot control events, you can be taught to govern your responses to them.

One of the body's normal responses to stress is increased secretion of hormones besides norepinephrine. In the chapter "Psychosomatic Factors and Tumor Growth" in *Risk Factors in Breast Cancer,* Dr. Basil Stoll cites research from the early seventies to show that emotional stress can affect the circulating levels of such pituitary-associated hormones as pro-lactin, growth hormone, gonadotropin, and corticotropin. Dr. Stoll concludes, "Of the pituitary trophic hormones which affect growth of established mammary cancer in humans, pro-lactin is considered the most important." This is why treatment for advanced breast cancer can involve not only removal of the ovaries but removal of the adrenal or pituitary glands as well.

Excessive corticosteroids produced under stress suppress the workings of the body's immune system and lower resistance to viruses and other disease producers. Changes in amine (nutrient) metabolism in the brain may create both mood disturbance and abnormalities in pituitary secretion.

A further biochemical response is discussed by Dr. A. Papaioannou in *Etiology of Human Breast Cancer*. Stress brings about the mobilization of free fatty acids, which are readily obtainable from fat deposits in the body. "Individuals with severe depressive illness often show elevated FFA (free fatty acids), and patients with cancer as a group have abnormally high FFA."

He cautions, however, that the relationship may be "only indirect." Excess free fatty acids presently remain another tantalizing biological marker that may someday provide an adequate test for early cancer.

Some work by Dr. V. Riley ("Mouse Mammary Tumors: Alteration of Incidence as Apparent Function of Stress," *Science,* 8/8/75, 465–67) is fascinating because through experimenting with various stresses on breast cancer-prone mice, he actually altered the incidence of the disease.

Mice of the C3H/HE strain typically develop cancer eight to eighteen months after birth from the mammary tumor virus transmitted in their milk. "Mammary tumor incidence at 400 days, however, was modified as a result of differential environmental stress conditions from 92 percent incidence under chronic stress to 7 percent incidence in the group provided a protected environment."

What constitutes stress to a female mouse, and how does she react? "The stress endured by mice in shipping, handling, and capturing produces typical stress reactions that ac-

tivate the adrenals, thus increasing concentrations of corticos-
terone." Such a concentration shrinks the thymus gland,
which in both young mice and humans influences the T-
lymphocyte cells that fight body invasion by foreign matter.

Corticoid influences may cause both an increase in MTV [mouse
tumor virus] production as well as an impairment in the immunological control of transformed cells. . . . It is further hypothe-
sized that once the cancer cell enters into a state which cannot be
handled by the limited defense abilities of immunological surveillance, the production of a fatal tumor becomes inevitable and is
nonreversible by natural host defenses.

That Dr. Riley, by controlling stress, reduced to 7 percent the incidence of breast cancer in a mouse strain that was
especially bred and fed to develop cancer is remarkable.

As such studies indicate, physical response to prolonged internal or external conflict can alter or destroy the
body's immunological effectiveness. Dr. George F. Solomon of
the Department of Psychiatry, School of Medicine, Stanford
University, gave a paper titled "Relationships among Cancer,
Emotions, Stress, and Immunity" at a Science Writers' Seminar sponsored by the American Cancer Society. First he re-
viewed four factors "found quite consistently in reports of
personality studies in some patients with cancer." They are:

- Loss of an important relationship prior to tumor development
    - Relative inability to express hostile feelings
    - Unresolved tension concerning a parental figure
    - Sexual problems.

He concluded:

These factors are very similar to those . . . I found in patients with
auto-immune diseases, particularly rheumatoid arthritis which, like
cancer, have been associated with relative deficiency of immunologic
responsivity. . . . There is growing evidence that resistance to cancer
is immunologic in nature. Some event reducing immunologic compe-
tence at a critical time may allow a mutant cell (ordinarily rejected
like a foreign graft) induced by virus, chemical carcinogen, radiation,
or chance somatic mutation to thrive and grow.

9 / The War on Viruses

Cancer can be prevented, yet we're spending more than $800 million looking for a cure and only about $20 million on prevention. We've been concentrating on two unyielding levels: (1) cancer treatment and (2) basic research that includes the vaccine program. After five years and a half billion dollars we have proved one thing: you cannot have a vaccine for cancer. —DR. IRWIN D. J. BROSS,
Director, Biostatistics, Roswell Park
Memorial Institute, Buffalo, New York.

More than 100 viruses, such as the Rous sarcoma virus, are now known to cause cancer in laboratory animals. Evidence for a human cancer virus—and hope for vaccine(s) against it—is presently incomplete or inadmissible, depending on which camp you question.

According to orthodox researchers, the only human tumor known by direct evidence to be virus-caused is warts.

An infectious virus has been defined as "a piece of bad news wrapped up in protein." It can live and reproduce only by entering a healthy cell, somehow inserting one or all of its genes into normal chromosomes, and ordering replication of itself using host nutrients. Since this process resembles the basic subversion involved in cancer, you can see why virus and vaccine research are funded and pursued, despite inconclusive results.

In the late thirties, Dr. Joseph Bittner at a Bar Harbor, Maine, laboratory isolated a virus responsible for breast cancer in some female mice. He was studying the effects of various crossbreedings of mice with low breast cancer incidence with mice of high incidence. He found that disease incidence in genetically identical members of the hybrid offspring groups differed according to how the parental strains were combined: mother with high incidence mated with father from a low-incidence strain, high-incidence father mated with low-incidence mother, etc. It was already known, of course, that the female parent had more influence than the male on production of mammary cancer. Although all offspring were genetically identical, they got breast cancer at differing rates, but these rates did not match the rates expected according to their parentage. One would suppose, for example, that offspring of high-incidence mothers and high-incidence fathers would all develop breast cancer and that few offspring of low-incidence parents would develop it. (No animal received hormone injections.)

Actual breast cancer figures for the offspring of various crossbreedings proved puzzlingly intermediate, implying some environmental factor from food or nursing which was affecting the rates. When Dr. Bittner removed the young from their mothers at birth and had them foster-nursed by mothers of another strain, these offspring later produced breast tumors at their foster mothers' rates, not at the expected rates of their biological mothers or fathers.

Bittner called the explanation "the milk factor." Finally, he isolated and identified it as an RNA (ribonucleic acid) virus of the B type ("B particle"). It is called MTV (mouse tumor virus) or MuMTV (murine mammary tumor virus). RNA viruses are thought to insinuate themselves into a cell and act as extra genes; DNA viruses tamper with the operations of normal genes already present.

It remains a sad puzzle that forty years' research has failed to identify an equivalent human breast cancer virus. "Viruslike particles" have been found in the breast milk of Parsi women in India. Since about half their cancer is breast cancer and they do breast-feed, they are the ethnic population most studied for breast cancer viruses. In 1969 different groups of researchers found B particles in some breast malignancies, in the milk of some women with breast cancer, and in 5 percent of the milk samples from healthy women. Thus no one can prove that these particles caused malignant tumors. They appear in some apparently healthy women—and do not appear in every breast cancer.

Bacteria, viruses, and cancer cells in the human body can produce what are called *antigens.* Tumor-associated antigens are specific proteins on the surface of cancer cells that betray their foreignness and should alert the immune system to produce *antibodies* to attack and kill them. (Some cells producing antibodies are called *lymphocytes.* Part of the immune response is achieved by two different classes of lymphoctyes: *B cells,* which bind to specific antigens, and *T cells,* which control larger scavenger cells, the *macrophages,* that fight and engulf whole microorganisms.) People like Eydie Mae (Chapter 6) who have a good tumor-host relationship must have immune systems that remain competent at fighting disease.

Part of the reason that cancer can overwhelm or evade the body's defenses may lie in a class of cells called *suppressor lymphocytes.* Discovered and announced in 1977 by the Sidney Farber Cancer Institute, Boston, these cells ordinarily monitor the immune response to assure that it continues to differentiate between "self" (normal cells, friendly bacteria) and "nonself" (harmful foreign matter). "You have to remember that the beauty of the immune system is that it doesn't respond to your own cells," remarked one researcher. So along with the fact that viruses live and reproduce hidden within previously normal cells, these suppressor lymphocytes may also camouflage what should be destroyed by other parts of the immune system. The process could involve "self" cells becoming cancerous independently or through action of an outside carcinogen, such as a virus.

Despite much recent work on immunotherapy (attempts to induce or increase body immunity to cancer), Dr. William Terry, associate director for immunology, Division of Cancer Biology, NCI, says: "An analysis of the development of clinical immunotherapy indicates that any illusions that immunotherapy would produce easy or dramatic solutions to the problems of cancer treatment were ill-founded. . . . Additional basic research as well as careful, time-consuming clinical studies will be required before immunotherapy can be established as a regular form of treatment for any human cancer."

Markers

An elevated amount of some body substance (hormone, enzyme, etc.) that might indicate the presence of cancer is called a *biological* or *biochemical marker.*

The search for markers specific to particular forms of cancer, including breast cancer, has proved frustrating. Dr. Morton K. Schwartz of Sloan-Kettering Institute (in response to a 1976 NIH request for a research proposal on "Longitudinal Studies of Biologic Markers in Breast Cancer Patients") reports:

The search for biochemical procedures useful in primary diagnosis and in following the course of metastatic breast cancer has not resulted in finding a single test or a combination of tests completely useful in this regard. . . . The analysis of carcinoembryonic antigen (CEA) has received the most attention. . . . [In one study] 45 percent of patients with breast cancer had elevated values. Abnormal values were seen in patients with other forms of cancer as well as individuals with a variety of benign diseases.

The author concludes, "The CEA test was found to be neither an efficient indicator of early metastatic disease nor an adequate test to monitor response to palliative therapy."

Under "Background of Work," this request states, "While no single marker thus far appears to be entirely specific for breast cancer, improved diagnostic specificity for breast cancer detection may be possible by using a number of such markers." This refers to work by Dr. Douglas Tormey (*Cancer* 35:1095, 1975).

In 1977 a new diagnostic test for breast cancer was announced. Named the *T-antigen test,* it is a skin test similar to that for tuberculosis and was devised from work with women who already had breast cancer. It is experimental and still under evaluation by Sloan-Kettering and its originator, Dr. George F. Springer, professor of microbiology and immunology at Northwestern University, Evanston, Illinois.

The test is based on the fact that cells of a breast tumor, no matter how small, produce T-antigen protein substances. The woman's immune system should respond to these substances with specific antibodies that lock onto these antigens and destroy the tumor cells. Although this does happen, some cells escape surveillance via a "blocking factor" mechanism; a tumor grows. Antibodies are present but are ineffective or otherwise unequal to the task.

When a small amount of such T-antigen is injected under a woman's skin, a local reaction—reddening or swelling—occurs about a day later only in those women who have breast cancer, even in an early (preclinical) stage. The test diagnoses those women whose systems have already tried to fight the disease with antibodies. Normal women test negative; that is, they have no reaction.

According to one report, the test detected breast cancer in seventy consecutive cases long before other cancer signs—lump, weight loss, pain—appeared.

Cryptocides and Immunotherapy

Dr. Virginia Livingston believes she has isolated the viruslike organism that causes cancer. With four other physicians, she practices medicine in San Diego, California.

It is a challenge to summarize in a few sentences her nearly forty years of research. Originally an internist, Livingston began in the 1940s to observe the bacilli that cause tuberculosis and leprosy. From there she moved to work with malignancies, and found in all she studied a virus organism she called *Cryptocides* ("hidden killer").

In her autobiography, *Cancer: A New Breakthrough,* she writes:

In 1947 I found a strange, many-formed, acid-fast [stains red under microscope after treatment with acid alcohol] organism present in all the cancers of animals and man studied. Until this time, although various kinds of cancer organism had been seen and described by many workers, their universal property of acid-fastness was not known. I also noted that they are extremely variable in size and shape but always have some forms that are acid-fast . . . which means that they can be identified and differentiated from other microbes that are not related to the cancer process.

She believes *Cryptocides* is latent in both humans and animals. In a random survey of 100 people, 40 percent presented blood from which it cultured rapidly; 20 percent cultured with difficulty, and 40 percent not at all. However, all cancer patients and those with collagen diseases (diseases of connective tissue, such as joints and bones) tested positive in one of her studies.

Here is part of a description titled "Darkfield Examination of Unstained Fresh Blood Preparation":

. . . pulsating orange bodies in the red cells may be observed. In the background, there are bright dancing forms which appear to be small L-forms of the organism. . . . Forms resembling a medusa or an octopus with waving filaments may be present. Organisms may bud from the surface of the red cells and form fine hairlike filaments which resemble the handle of a tennis racquet. . . .

Changes in the character of the leukocytes [white blood cells] are also apparent. Many leukocytes in the advanced stage of disease appear smudged, inactive, and only dimly luminescent whereas normal leukocytes have vigorously active granules and active amoeboid movements.

To Dr. Livingston, cancer is a failure of the immune system. She has devised vaccines she considers effective against cancer; she combines them with other therapy. For each patient, her staff prepares an individualized "autogenous" vaccine from organisms in the urine, which are cultured, killed, then injected into the patient. She uses this along with gamma globulin (the protein part of blood plasma that contains antibodies), standard antibiotics, small doses of chemotherapy where necessary, and attention to diet (vitamins, enzymes). In her book she describes the progress and remission of several breast cancer cases.

In 1972, after publishing several articles on *Cryptocides* in medical journals, she presented her work and methods to the American Cancer Society's Seminar for Science Writers. There was no large response, since she was not affiliated with any major research organization. And she was daring to treat human beings without a large-scale animal trial of her vaccines.

In 1977, testing finally began. Cooperation with a Japanese researcher produced an improved vaccine to be used on 1,200 mice at Harvard. Early results seem favorable. Cancer cells injected into vaccinated mice grew in only 10 percent to 20 percent of the animals; about 80 percent appeared protected.

Many years ago doctors noted that patients who survived either tuberculosis or leprosy did not get cancer in middle or old age. Fighting those disease organisms somehow provided immunity to cancer, just as milkmaids who had had cowpox were immune to smallpox, a fact noted by Edward Jenner in 1796.

If only *all* cancer were a virus . . .

So far, orthodox medicine suspects viruses are involved in only two forms of cancer—Hodgkin's disease and Burkitt's lymphoma—because evidence of geographical "hot spots" for these two cancers shows up on epidemiological maps. Further research will probably prove Dr. Livingston correct—viruses cause some cancers, even some breast cancer, but cannot account for the total incidence of the disease or the fact that not everyone exposed gets the disease. There again we must look to heredity, hormones, and other predisposing or promoting factors.

I attended a program on international cancer research that included a talk and slides by Dr. Eberhard Wecker, director of the Institute for Virus Research, University of Würzburg, West Germany. Part of the institute's work involves immunobiological experiments with tumor viruses causing fowl leukemia. Mortality rates from these viruses can actually be altered—decreased two-thirds—by protective antiserum injections given within nine days after infection. However, even in infectious leukemia of mice, viruses must be *injected;* sharing a cage with an infected animal is insufficient to spread this leukemia.

It is now thought that human beings inherit a variety of endogenous viruses (those originating within the body). Ordinarily they remain dormant inside cells and do not migrate or reproduce. Possibly these viruses mediate or help activate the immune response against harmful viruses coming from outside. Their purpose may also be to assure the slight differentiation of genetic material in daughter cells following mitosis (cell division). A selection of different viruses among the genes of cells could assure basic adaptability at the microscopic level, and therefore strengthen the whole organism. A crude analogy would be to an organization that prospers with individuals of differing abilities.

According to Dr. Wecker, cancer would be "a pathological mutation of this normal process of viral expression." Since it can involve viruses, genes, processes already within the body's definition of "self," the immune system is not primed to fight what it has no reason to perceive as an invader.

Several speakers on the program repeated the prevailing wisdom of contemporary viral research: "So far, *no* human virus has been found to cause cancer. These viruses are in humans, but they have *not* been incriminated. The people are normal."

One of the "in jokes" of viral research parodies what are known as *Koch's postulates* (microorganism must be present in all cases, must produce the disease in susceptible animals, must be identifiable and recoverable at any point):

> *Four Easy Steps to Nobel Prize:*
> Plug virus into cell; wait 3.25 days.
> Harvest virus.
> Immunize mouse with virus.
> Add virus-induced cancer cells to mouse.
> *Voilà*—immunity. CURE. Nobel Prize!

10/ A "Cancer Epidemic"?

I wouldn't say we're making tremendous headway, but we are making some progress. The improvement in the more common cancers—breast, colon, lungs—has not been as dramatic as in the leukemia and lymphoma types. . . . I do agree not enough has been spent on prevention. American medicine has tended to traditionally train people for diagnosis and treatment. —DR. ARTHUR C. UPTON,
Director, NCI

What if decades ago we tried to cure infectious disease by treating each sick individual instead of creating political support for plumbing and sanitation? That's where we are with cancer. It's a preventable disease. —DR. SIDNEY WOLFE,
Director, Public Citizens'
Health Research Group, Washington, D.C.

We knew 20 years ago that many of these pesticides caused cancer in animals, yet there was relatively little research about their potential for harm until recently. I think this has to be the coverup of the century in health. —DR. ROBERT MOBBS,
member, Massachusetts Pesticides Board

Drs. Glenn Paulson and Peter Preuss have estimated that 60 to 90 percent of cancer is attributable to environmental factors. This includes the whole range of known or suspected carcinogens, such as tars from smoking combined with alcohol use, high-cholesterol diet, radiation, specific occupational hazards, drugs, pesticides, and other chemicals. A recent tabloid newspaper article claimed that nine-tenths of cancer was immediately preventable, and suggested that somebody—probably the American Cancer Society—should be sued when next year's statistics appear.

Few can deny by this time that the U.S. economy, born in Western frontier psychology and sharing errors common to industrialized countries, has based itself on squandering resources and neglecting the resultant pollution. For example, Lake Erie is the only body of water on earth that's a fire hazard because it's drowning in chemicals.

Federal control of known or suspected carcinogens is fragmented among at least five agencies and a welter of laws. These agencies and their specific responsibilities are shown in Figure 6.

Figure 6. FEDERAL AGENCIES CONTROLLING KNOWN
OR SUSPECTED CARCINOGENS

AGENCY	JURISDICTION
Food and Drug Administration	2,500 food additives 20,000 prescription drugs 300,000 patent remedies 4,000 chemicals for cosmetics
Environmental Protection Agency	35,000 pesticides Investigation of air and water pollution
Occupational Health and Safety Administration	20,000 chemical compounds in industry
Consumer Product Safety Administration	10,000 products in 350 categories involving about half of all U.S. businesses
Nuclear Regulatory Commission	Safety of atomic energy plants Nuclear reactors for industrial research

Obviously this division of responsibility spells confusion and delay in effective control, even assuming that research into the harmful effects of any substance is honestly done and reported. Remember that no research can guarantee anything as "totally safe." All it can do is state that with the particular amounts tested under particular laboratory conditions, certain harmful effects were or were not observed.

One congressional study noted, "The fragmentation of research and control—largely taken in response to newly discovered hazard—can be expected to continue. At issue is whether this largely ad hoc, fragmented policy can adequately protect health and the environment in today's advanced society."

In the laboratory, not only can the same carcinogen, such as coal tars, produce different kinds of tumors but the same kind of tumor can be induced by different carcinogens. In *The Nature of Cancer,* P. M. Sutton, a British professor and researcher, wrote:

It is of considerable theoretical importance that the same carcinogen can produce completely different tumors depending on its site of action. For example, benzpyrene [a coal tar derivative] on the skin will produce squamous cell carcinoma; under the skin it induces sarcoma of fibrous tissue. But these are two completely different cancers . . . under the microscope . . . [and] in naked eye appearance and behavior. . . . For most cancers, the cause is not known; and yet the same cause (e.g., benzpyrene) can produce different tumors . . . while, conversely, the same tumor (e.g., squamous cell carcinoma) can be induced by quite different agents, including various chemical carcinogens and X rays.

Dr. Elizabeth Whelan, a specialist in public health and executive director of the American Council of Science and Health, urges a more balanced view of environmental dangers. She wrote me:

It is my concern that Americans are unnecessarily worked up about "environmental carcinogens," having arrived at the conclusion that we are surrounded by a virtual army of noxious chemicals. In a sense this is a somewhat comforting view for many people to take, in that it relieves them of the responsibility for cancer prevention—it is all industry's fault.

Looking at epidemiological trends, it is clear that (a) there is no cancer epidemic in this country—the epidemic is solely limited to lung cancer. If it were not for lung cancer, the cancer death rate in this country would have been stable or declining for the past 30 years; (b) there is no reason to believe that we are being victimized by cancer-causing agents around us. Other than the rare cases (e.g., occupational cancers which account for some 3 percent maximum of cancer deaths), the causes of cancer are either within our control (cigarette smoking, imprudent diet, excessive sun exposure) or unknown.

I think it is a pity that people are worrying about food additives, when they should be more concerned about the other 99.9999 percent of the food they eat—and the link of *that* and cancer risk.

She is correct that the media tend to concentrate on certain newsworthy scare substances—nitrites, asbestos, saccharin, pesticides, red dye #2, DES hormone to fatten cattle. And this overfocus induces either fatalism (there is *nothing* one can do against the plague of unknowns and semiknowns) or paranoia (*everything* causes cancer). Dr. Whelan pointed out other facts not generally known: a small amount of nitrite is a natural component of human saliva, and estrogen occurs naturally in wheat germ, unpolished rice, some vegetable oils, honey, and some legumes (beans).

One can argue over a definition of "epidemic." Even if we take into account the fact that the present numerical increase in cancer cases is partly due to more people living longer, having avoided the infectious diseases of previous centuries, still the statistic that one-quarter of Americans will get some form of cancer represents an incalculable amount of human suffering.

While there is no known safe level of exposure to some carcinogenic substances or processes (for example, radiation), most researchers agree it is *repeated exposure* that causes cancer. In Carlton Fredericks' words:

It seems to me unlikely that one wrong molecule may cause cancer; if that were true, I doubt I'd be here to write these lines, or you to read them. We've all, knowingly or unknowingly, ingested *billions* of wrong molecules; every woman has, who has taken an estrogen-based birth control pill or used lipstick containing a carcinogenic red dye. If you've eaten a licorice candy, you've swallowed a cancer-producing black coloring. If you've enjoyed a barbecued steak, you've displayed a yen for the taste which comes from the breakdown products of heated animal fats, known to be at least cocarcinogenic.

There are commonsense, although difficult, home or daily life measures to take against cancer like quitting cigarette smoking, changing your diet, and avoiding unnecessary X rays, including mammography if you have no suspicious symptoms like a lump or sudden loss of weight and you are under fifty. Fear of unknown carcinogens should not prevent you from paying attention to known or suspected ones.

In the late sixties, Dr. E. Cuyler Hammond, currently ACS vice president for epidemiology and statistics, and other researchers at Mt. Sinai School of Medicine, Manhattan, published data showing that the lung cancer rate in asbestos workers who smoke a pack or more a day is ninety-two times that of nonsmokers or of nonworkers with asbestos. (The lung cancer rate for all asbestos workers is seven times that of the general population.) It is logical to conclude that smoking has a multiplier effect on other risk factors.

Although the Johns Manville Company reduced airborne asbestos fiber levels, it was early 1978 before the company banned smoking in all asbestos units—14 locations employing 8,000 workers—and introduced nonsmoking clinics.

Certainly, we must continue the drive to end environmental pollution and test potential carcinogens, but right now women can do a great deal on their own to reduce personal risk.

"Lies, Damned Lies, and Statistics"

The techniques used in statistical research into breast cancer—or any disease, for that matter—are complicated, but it is important to understand what the statistics mean.

For any disease, incidence rates (morbidity) exceed death rates (mortality). Because communities, countries, and continents vary in population size, the incidence or deaths in a given year are best expressed by percentages or rates—numbers per 100,000 population—rather than by absolute numbers.

For example, the number of new cases of female breast cancer in the United States for 1978 is estimated to be approximately 91,000. The *crude rate* of newly diagnosed female breast cancer in the United States, estimated for 1978 in women age twenty-one and over, is approximately .13 percent. That's about ⅛ of 1 percent. It amounts to one in 780 women yearly (approximately 71,000,000 women age twenty-one and over divided by 91,000 new breast cancer cases; 1976 *Statistical Abstract of the United States* population figure).

Since a crude rate for incidence covers all ages or age groups, you can get much more information from a set of rates for specific age groups. The annual *age-specific* incidence *rate* is the number of cases occurring at a given age or age range divided by the number achieving that age or age range during the year.

Figure 7. ANNUAL AGE-SPECIFIC U.S. INCIDENCE
RATES OF BREAST CANCER PER 100,000
FEMALE POPULATION

AGE	NUMBER PER 100,000 OF THE AGE GROUP	EQUIVALENT PERCENT
20–24	1.1	.001
. . .		. . .
80–84	301.3	.30

Note: The final number is not 30 percent but ³/₁₀ of 1 percent. For the whole table containing these numbers, see Figures 8 and 9. Age-specific percentages, for instance, are less than the overall crude rate (.13 percent) up to approximately age forty-four; they are higher after that age.

Because death rates and incidence rates vary widely according to age levels, comparing two countries or two widely separated time periods where the age distributions in the population are radically different can be misleading. The so-called annual *standardized* death or incidence *rate* is computed from age-specific rates of each country applied to the distribution of ages in an arbitrarily selected or hypothetical country. These results, too, vary according to the standard chosen.

For example, the crude incidence rate for stomach cancer in urban males in Norway in 1970 was 38 per 100,000. The standardized incidence rate was 25.3 per 100,000. Or, to compare countries with high and low rates of female breast

Figure 8. U.S. BREAST CANCER INCIDENCE FOR
DIFFERENT AGE GROUPINGS OF WOMEN

AVERAGE ANNUAL AGE-SPECIFIC INCIDENCE
RATES PER 100,000 POPULATION

AGE	INCIDENCE	PERCENTAGE OF WOMEN
15–19	—	—
20–24	1.1	0.001
25–29	8.7	0.009
30–34	22.5	0.02
35–39	52.5	0.05
40–44	103.7	0.10
45–49	159.2	0.16
50–54	171.7	0.17
55–59	191.8	0.19
60–64	226.2	0.23
65–69	234.2	0.23
70–74	259.8	0.26
75–79	294.9	0.30
80–84	301.3	0.30
85+	307.9	0.31

(SOURCE: Third National Cancer Survey, Monograph 41, National Institutes of Health, S. J. Cutler and J. L. Young, editors, 1975.)

cancer incidence: Switzerland's (Geneva) age-standardized incidence rate of the disease was 96.5 cases per 100,000 and Japan's (average of three tumor registries), 18.2 cases per 100,000 (*Cancer Incidence in Five Continents,* 1976, figures standardized to a European population).

A *competing* health or death *risk* is the statistical chance that a person with cancer will get or die of another disease within a given time period. A woman age eighty-five, for example, treated for breast cancer, is likely to die of something else before her cancer recurs or metastasizes. One reason that breast cancer is the leading killer in women age forty to forty-four is that competing risks (death from childbirth, stroke, heart disease, etc.) are low during those years.

It is as easy to manipulate data in breast cancer research and treatment as it is in other fields by selecting for a treatment project, for instance, only those women with minimal cancer likely to do well whatever therapy is chosen and

Figure 9. U.S. BREAST CANCER INCIDENCE
SHOWN AS A LINE GRAPH

ANNUAL AGE-SPECIFIC INCIDENCE RATES
PER 100,000 POPULATION

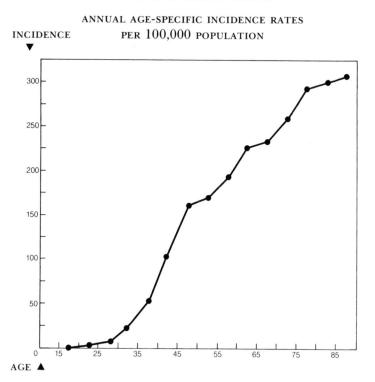

(SOURCE: Third National Cancer Survey, Monograph 41, National Institutes of Health, S. J. Cutler and J. L. Young, editors, 1975.)

excluding those with extensive nodal involvement or other signs that spell poor prognosis.

One example, which is important because such research determines whether women lose or save their breasts, was given during the 1976 congressional hearings into breast cancer. Dr. Vincent DeVita, director of NCI Division of Cancer Treatment, refuted part of Dr. Cushman Haagensen's defense of radical mastectomy by stating:

Those surgeons who select patients for "operability" and small tumors, with no or few axillary glands involved, will have the best results whatever operation is used; but their results may be irrelevant in regard to the universe of patients with breast cancer. . . .

In all the reports cited by Dr. Haagensen, including his own, biases enter into and influence the interpretation of the data. For example, Dr. Haagensen uses his population of patients who had biopsy proven disease in the internal mammary and/or supraclavicular lymph gland chain (who received radiotherapy as the primary treatment *instead of* surgery) as an example of the ineffectiveness of radiotherapy as a primary treatment. Here he now uses survival as his guidepost. The data he presents are misleading. Survival *is* bad in this group in Dr. Haagensen's study, as one would expect. The patients had proven glandular disease which, as I have said, reflects the presence of distant metastases. The survival of these patients *would have been equally bad had they had a radical mastectomy;* wasn't this the reason he excluded them from consideration for radical mastectomy in the first place? It is not fair, then, to use these survival data to reflect negatively on the potential effectiveness of radiotherapy, *to control the local tumor,* after excisional biopsy, in a group ineligible for surgery by his own criteria.

The Risk of Risks

One aim of breast cancer research is to calculate future probable risks for groups of women sharing one or more characteristics that are known or suspected to affect incidence. The American Cancer Society has estimated that 80 percent of American women age thirty to fifty have at least one risk factor in their personal histories although only 7 percent—one in thirteen—actually get the disease during their life span.

Remember that probabilities are statistically determined based on retrospective data. While they are applicable to general populations, their prospective (predictive) use for the individual woman is limited.

Even if you fall into one of the highest risk groups—daughter of a mother with breast cancer, for instance—no one, including your doctor, can predict whether the disease will strike *you.* Examine your breasts regularly and keep informed about the disease. Should you find a lump, neither ignore it nor assume the worst. Eight of ten lumps (another statistical average!) are benign.

This "race after risk factors" has its black-humor side. Two ingenious researchers sat down one day and invented what has to be the epidemiologist's dream woman (H. P. Leis and A. Raciti, "The Search for Women at High Risk" in Stoll, *Risk Factors for Breast Cancer*). Now that you have read about diet, hormones, heredity, psychological factors, viruses, and environment, can you guess who she is?

The search for the patient with the highest risk of developing breast cancer would culminate in the finding of a fifty-one-year-old fat, hypothyroid Caucasian nun, living in a cold climate in the Western hemisphere, with a wet type of cerumen [ear wax] and a prolonged menstrual history, whose mother and sister had premenopausal bilateral breast cancer, who was nursed by a mother who had B-viral particles in her milk, who has had endometrial cancer and a cancer in one breast, whose random biopsy of the other breast showed a precancerous mastopathy, who has a low estriol fraction and an abnormal Bulbrook discriminant, who is immunodeficient, who received heavy radiation exposure during treatment for TB by repeated fluoroscopies, and who has a high dietary fat intake.

Luckily this unfortunate creature remains a fantasy—*too* perfect an example of pathological predestination to exist in the real world.

11 / A Case in Point

Researchers in biophysics, as distinct from biochemistry or endocrinology, have developed their own theory of cancer causation. Some of this work—and a typical response to it—illustrates how the truth about cancer arrives in spurts, fragmented, relative to the different specialties pursuing it. It also exists *beyond* any of them, or the Nobel Prize for the "answer to cancer" would have been awarded years ago.

You probably recall the tale of the blind philosophers. Each touched a different part of the same elephant, so one philosopher reported that "elephantness" consisted of a trunk, another of a tail, another a rough hide, etc. Nobody comprehended—therefore everybody ignored—the total animal. One response to the following biophysical theory of cancer shows the myopia of some entrenched minds currently performing cancer research.

Dr. Fritz Popp is a German chemist and professor of radiology who has staked his professional reputation on a theory of cancer as a form of disturbed communication among cells—"impaired biosignals." The components of body cells, like all electron particles of matter (according to the wave theory of physics), are in constant, if minute, motion. This helps generate body heat and even light. The much photographed Kirelian aura around some people's bodies is an example. Differential areas of body heat constitute the physical principle behind thermography to detect breast tumors.

Cancer cells in a tumor show up as "hot spots" on heat-sensitive paper.

According to the radiation theory, it is disturbed communication, misused electromagnetic energy, that results in tumor growth and invasion. Dying cells emit much stronger radiation than healthy ones; dead cells are those with no radiant energy left.

Utilizing sunlight, biophysical processes provide the primal energy that directs human biochemistry and physiology (metabolism of food and hormones; production of enzymes; growth and repair of tissue). Local control of these processes occurs via genes within the chromosomes of each body cell. According to Dr. Popp's theory, biophysics is really a higher order of reality controlling biochemistry.

However, biochemists—and 99 percent of current cancer research is biochemical—either do not condone or ignore such a professional challenge. After I'd read Dr. Popp's book in German (the possible English title is *How Cancer Could Develop*), I discussed it with a cancer researcher knowledgeable about international work on cancer. His response was somewhere between hysteria and apoplexy: "The man is mad! What he's done is a schizophrenic production!" The usual contentions followed: Dr. Popp, besides being deranged, must be fraudulent; must have fudged his data, testing effects of light on dishes of normal and cancerous cells separated by a quartz barrier; was at best misguided; etc.

Next I received a retelling of the (in)famous French experiment with colored and white ducklings—insult by analogy. The mystery of how white eggs, injected with cells (not sperm) from colored ducks, produced colored ducklings was finally solved when somebody, probably the janitor, noticed a colored drake had flown over the fence and was courting the white ducks.

And Dr. Popp is no charlatan prescribing lemon juice for terminal cancer. His ideas stem from years of work in theoretical radiology.

I do not discuss his work in order to vindicate him by attacking his attackers. I cite his case as one example of the politics of medical/scientific research, which ought to ask, "Is it true?" or "How does it work?" but asks first or instead, "Is he crazy?" and "How much money did they give him?"

DIAGNOSING AND TREATING

12 / Natalia: Awaiting the Verdict

Natalia had the surgeon every woman dreads—the one who ignores her initial symptom, a malignant breast lump, until surgery, when finally done, is a full radical mastectomy.

And Natalia became the patient every doctor dreads—the one so enraged by medical negligence and damage to her work life that she sues for malpractice. Of 91,000 women diagnosed with breast cancer yearly, the majority still undergo some form of mastectomy with emotions that range from willingness to horror. Natalia is one who fought to save her breast until the last moment.

Natalia is an artist, film maker, and language teacher who lives in Manhattan. Besides these talents, she has also danced professionally with various companies. I interviewed her in her loft studio near one of her paintings—a self-portrait of a strong, black-haired woman with partial draping around two full breasts. Natalia now remarks of such work, "When I got out of the hospital, I was devastated physically, psychologically. I had dreams that I'd actually died. I didn't even recognize photos of myself or work I did before the radical mastectomy. After that, nothing was the same."

In August 1972, Natalia found a lump she described as "lima-bean sized" in her right breast toward the breastbone. Since she believed her own physician, Dr. B., was retiring after nearly forty years as one of New York's leading surgeons and author of research papers on breast cancer treatment, she first had mammography and palpation at a clinic specializing in this. Because she was in her mid-thirties, the clinic staff asked her to return after her next menstrual period.

Following the second visit, she also saw Dr. B. He had biopsied two benign tumors when she was twenty-three and thirty-one years old, and he was familiar with her case, diagnosed as benign fibrocystic disease. A condition that affects about 50 percent of U.S. women at some point in their lives, it is most common in premenopausal women. Specialists disagree whether and to what extent it may predispose to breast cancer.

While palpating the breast, Dr. B. cradled it in his hand to demonstrate what Natalia already knew—the tumor had fixated itself to the skin, a serious indication for malignancy. Although fibrocystic breasts may feel generally lumpy, neither Dr. B. nor the radiologist who had analyzed the mammograms indicated at this point any lump other than that fixated in the right breast. Another radiologist later reported that these mammograms had been misfocused, and therefore were useless for diagnosis.

When Natalia indicated to Dr. B. that she hoped he would perform a lumpectomy, as he had done on the previous occasions, he scheduled a hospital biopsy. (Biopsy excises the lump plus a safe margin of surrounding tissue.) The hospital's examining physician corroborated Dr. B.'s finding of a single lump.

Natalia's first indication of something irregular came as she was wheeled into the operating room. Dr. B. asked, "Which breast is it?"—a question unlikely to reassure a tense patient, whether or not she has signed the consent form allowing mastectomy. He had neither visited her room before surgery nor taken her chart into the operating room.

Next she remembered him at her side the following day saying, "You're all right." She felt bandages on the opposite, right, side of the right breast (toward the arm), 180 degrees *away from* the original lump. After two days in the hospital she returned home. She lost some weeks of teaching while the incision healed.

However, the original lump was still there.

She soon questioned Dr. B. about it. He answered that during surgery he had found a second, larger, and presumably more dangerous tumor which he had removed from that right side of the right breast. Natalia was shocked and bewildered: why had he ignored an obvious, fixated lump to remove another that nobody but him had spotted?

He replied, "That first lump got smaller. I took out the one that would have given you trouble. You'll never have cancer." When she again referred to it, he asked, "Why do you keep talking about that lump?" implying that he had removed the only lump that, although benign, was possibly precancerous.

To me, Natalia insisted, "If he had been honest and said, 'That other lump is still dangerous. I intend to remove it,' I would have understood, even if it meant another biopsy.

"Part of me wanted to believe him." However, she sensed he was lying to her, and she was outraged at his removing a benign lump no one else had seen, to the neglect of a probably cancerous one. Furthermore, he had evaded her questions and attempted to deny his failure or poor judgment.

Determined to sue him for endangering her life, she obtained the name of a Manhattan law firm that specializes in malpractice suits. She contends her consent form had given him permission to remove *all* lumps found, including especially the cancerous one. The only way Dr. B. could justify ignoring the cancerous lump would be if he believed it benign. His later, pretrial defense postulated, however, that he had intended to watch and remove it but was prevented by the fact that Natalia had consented and probably would consent only to biopsy, not to mastectomy. If he made another hospital reservation for more surgery on Natalia, "None of this was said or phoned to me," she stated.

A woman who has already endured three lumpectomies without need of mastectomy may not easily see the need for mastectomy at all, even should cancer be found. Certainly radical mastectomy, whether standard or modified, "seemed like the equivalent of having my arm removed because of a splinter in my finger," to quote Win Ann Winkler, author of *Post-Mastectomy*. Nor is a woman with benign disease, who is used to negotiating forms and procedures, easily intimidated by medical personnel.

Armed with knowledge that cancer is a systemic disease, that mastectomy, no matter how radical, will not cure all women, and that surgeons like Dr. Oliver Cope and others (Chapter 15) believe lumpectomy, followed by irradiation or chemotherapy as needed, cures just as many, some women in the late 1970s are refusing consent to any mastectomy. In 1972, however, Natalia was not fated to be one of these.

"I knew I had to get another doctor," she remarked, but after the first hospitalization costs, "I was broke." In November 1972 she did pursue further treatment, another exam and mammograms, at a Manhattan hospital that specializes in cancer care. About the lump Dr. B. had failed to remove, she saw written on the new mammography form: "Suspected malignancy."

Knowing the pressure toward mastectomy would now mount, she again negotiated for lumpectomy. A female radiologist on the staff wrote a three-page letter explaining Natalia's reasons, professional and personal. To me, Natalia said, "I feel this surgery is a medieval thing."

During a 1976 congressional subcommittee hearing, Rose Kushner, also a mastectomee, testified, "From what I have read of Dr. William Stewart Halsted [nineteenth-century American surgeon who pioneered mastectomy], I'm sure that if he were alive today, he would be the first person to put the mastectomy that bears his name on the museum shelf next to the leech."

However, Natalia's new surgeon, Dr. C., again a man of years' experience and research, turned hostile at the mere thought of a woman with suspected malignancy rejecting the standard treatment, some form of radical mastectomy. Finally he screamed at her, *before* even biopsying the lump, "You're stupid if you don't let me take your breast off. Only whores want to hold onto their breasts."

Natalia commented, "The whole atmosphere reeked of You're-a-bad-little-girl-not-doing-what-Daddy-tells-you. He was brutal in a professional way: we're doing this for your own good. They're boys on white chargers against disease, and anybody who disagrees is a whore. He made it into a sexual, instead of a medical, topic." Of Dr. C.'s personal motivation for temper tantrums related to his favorite surgery, Natalia added, "His mother died of breast cancer because, according to him, she refused to have a mastectomy. So he goes around saving the world by chopping off women's breasts!"

Finally Natalia and Dr. C. compromised; he would biopsy the lump under general anesthesia before, and only with her consent, proceeding further. In the hospital he visited her room and again "screamed at me." As she emerged from surgery on December 14, 1972, he was there stating, "You have cancer, my dear. Are you going to let me do the right thing now?"

The "right thing" meant, of course, mastectomy, since he apparently neither used nor admitted any alternate effective treatment for someone of Natalia's age. When Natalia refused consent, Dr. C. told her brother-in-law, a psychiatrist whose aid and concern supported her throughout, that lumpectomy has only a 30 percent survival rate "while we have a 90 percent survival rate." Without mastectomy he predicted she would die.

I was unable to ascertain the exact size or kind of tumor she had beyond the report that it was "infiltrating with triangular features"—facts upon which the doctor must have based his dire prediction. In his case, such facts appear to be secondary to his belief that any breast cancer (except perhaps the largest, ulcerating kind, rarely seen now) necessitates mastectomy. Under pressure, Natalia's brother-in-law finally promised to aid Dr. C. in forcing her consent.

She remarked bitterly, "I wasn't told of the options, even that there were any."

Meanwhile her legal case against the first doctor was proceeding. In a radio interview, Barbara Seaman and Dr. Gideon Seaman, authors of *Women and the Crisis in Sex Hormones,* observed, "A patient isn't likely to sue a doctor who has treated her as an adult, let her participate in decision making, warned her about possible side effects." Natalia lacked the good fortune to encounter such a physician, at least among her surgeons.

On December 18, 1972, Dr. C. performed a full (Halsted) radical mastectomy. He stated that the cancer's adherence to the chest muscles justified their removal. To Natalia's brother-in-law, however, Dr. C. admitted that none of the underarm lymph nodes, also removed, proved cancerous. She spent a total of ten days in the hospital and described the nursing care as generally good.

She doubts that either the full radical procedure or the series of radiation treatments that followed was necessary. She believes the radical surgery in particular was chosen to teach her a lesson about submissive conduct befitting a female patient in a doctor's presence.

The deep incision that channels across her chest, into the armpit, up to the collarbone, is visible under everything but the loosest clothing. She was unable to return to work for several months. When she did return, "I'd come in holding onto the desk and chair to get through the day." Luckily she had a sympathetic male department chairman who kept her job open.

In April 1973, Natalia's brother-in-law fought with Dr. C., trying to convince him to sign the medical disability forms that would allow her sick-leave insurance coverage to continue.

When I inquired what other help she received from family or friends, she smiled. "They called, came, and wrote. My brother-in-law called every night of the hospital stay." Natalia's mother arrived to assist with home care. "My mother is just a saint." At first Natalia, like other mastectomees, wouldn't look at herself or bathe without a towel around her chest. Finally her mother pulled the towel away one day, uttering the Yiddish equivalent of "Big deal!" She and her daughter laughed for almost the first time during her recovery period.

"People can make me laugh at it," Natalia continued. One of her circle of artistic friends even remarked of the one-breastedness, "In Berlin of the twenties you'd have been a sensation!"

A woman psychologist in a co-counseling group assisted Natalia in private sessions. Natalia described her as "very supportive and beautiful."

Every mastectomee, however, is ultimately alone with

her own terror at what has occurred and the knowledge that she has had cancer. "My best friends came—and left. It's a death trip. I felt they came and laid flowers on my tomb." Her boyfriend also arrived at the hospital. Although he denied feeling overwhelmed by what had befallen Natalia, he saw her less and less. Like Elise (Chapter 14), she was willing to speak frankly about the effect of mastectomy on her private life. "I can't be touched around the breast anywhere. I can't enjoy sex anymore. Men like you after mastectomy for all the wrong reasons. They think you'll be more willing to accept them, and you're not into doing *anything!*"

Although she did buy a comfortable breast prosthesis, no amount of padding can conceal or repair her deformed shoulder and underarm area.

She described the devastation that mastectomy has caused to her professional life, both physically and socially. "My arm still has limited motion, and I can't hold a camera." Her films done in the early seventies are shown in Manhattan and at schools and museums around the United States and Europe.

Competition in the arts is fierce. She feels some colleagues used the occasion of her illness to attack her work and exclude her from shows where she would normally have exhibited her paintings or films. Although in 1972 she'd received a grant, during her convalescence she could not assemble the work, records, and references needed to reapply. She lost her chance at a grant in 1973.

Concerning the total medical experience, she concluded, "You really feel death. I was an intense, heated, passionate person. Now I have to keep myself at a much lower level."

Finally we discussed her million-dollar suit against Dr. B. and the impending trial. First his lawyer questioned and examined her. Next, in the presence of her lawyer, the opposition's psychiatrist and physician both examined her. Finally came several sessions with a psychiatrist who would testify in her behalf at the trial. Dr. B. offered $10,000 for an out-of-court settlement. She refused, believing that five months' unnecessary coexistence with cancer plus five years' wait for a court date in New York City's crowded judicial apparatus justified the public event of a trial. If the case is decided in her favor, she hopes to recover enough money to pay court costs and the fee for whatever plastic surgery can do to restore the appearance of her scarred breast and shoulder area. By early 1978 the case was due to begin trial.

According to a 1977 poll done by NBC for a television special titled "Medicine in America: Life, Death, and Dollars," 7 percent of several thousand Americans queried said they had seriously considered suing one of their doctors. Anesthesiologists and surgeons are the specialists most often sued.

Regarding her own case, Natalia feels that any person who is a dancer has a heightened relationship to her body as a medium for expression of vitality and feeling. A painter requires a similar sense of joy and beauty in her own body and the human form. A prime horror for any creative person is to be forced to spend any portion of life in numbness or apathy, since artworks should spring from events felt with depth and love.

Natalia remarked, "After the surgery, nothing was the same, neither pleasure nor deep pain. It was such a great trauma, confronting the fact of my mutilation. The only way I do as well as I do is to deny the whole thing."

13 / Saving Breast and Life: New Diagnostic Methods

A woman named Joy—a friend of a friend—called me late one winter evening. Mammography, taken during her annual physical exam, had revealed three suspicious spots in the upper outer quadrant of the left breast. Too small to be felt, they showed on the mammogram as tiny white areas ("really millimeter-sized") of suspected calcification. Some malignant tumors attract calcium, which makes them hard when felt. What her mammogram showed could not yet be felt.

She already had one surgeon who would perform a biopsy by staining the questionable tissue inside the breast with special dyes to assure that all the suspected but probably invisible (to the naked eye) malignancy got removed through a small skin incision. She also had a general practitioner and a radiologist, both women.

At this point, the surgeon was not pressuring her toward mastectomy for such minimal cancer—if, indeed, it was cancer. She wanted to learn what I knew about the reliability and availability of other diagnostic procedures besides mammography and about the use of irradiation following a lumpectomy or partial mastectomy.

I was pleased to see that she had assembled her own medical-care team of practitioners who seemed concerned and negotiable—willing to explain the various possibilities without terrifying her.

When I asked, "Will you tell me your age?" she replied, "Postmenopausal."

I then told her that mammography was indeed performing its task of revealing suspicious tissue areas where nothing abnormal was yet palpable. Such a minimal breast cancer has the best possible chance of being localized to the breast, and therefore is most amenable to surgery, radiotherapy, or whatever treatment combination is indicated or negotiated.

Mammography

Mammography is an X-ray process now recommended yearly for all women age fifty or over. Guidelines issued in 1977 restrict its use in younger women to:

• Those age thirty-five through thirty-nine with a personal history of breast cancer, and
• Those age forty through forty-nine with either a personal or a family history of breast cancer in first-degree relatives (mother or sister).

Before its widespread recent use on 280,000 women in the Breast Cancer Detection Demonstration Project (BCDDP), mammography's effectiveness, especially in locating minimal cancer, was proved through the HIP (Health Insurance Plan of New York) screening plan begun in 1963. Sixty-two thousand women, age forty to sixty-four, were divided into study and control groups. At one point Dr. Philip Strax, medical director of Guttman Breast Diagnostic Institute, Manhattan, reported, "The results of a six-year follow-up of all women showed a remarkable reduction in the number of deaths from breast cancer in the study group compared with those in the control group. The one-third reduction in mortality persisted into the seventh year of follow-up."

At five years, 70 percent of the patients whose cancers were detected by mammography were free of metastases. The comparable figure for the control group (those who received medical care but not mammography) was only 46 percent.

Few doubt the need or value of mammography for older or high-risk women. As with any diagnostic tool, particularly one involving radiation, however, there are problems. Rose Kushner has publicized the fact that very few of the nation's 5,000 to 6,000 radiotherapy units, including mammography equipment, are monitored or calibrated regularly by NCI. Ralph Nader's Health Research Group obtained data on fifty-seven X-ray machines used in the BCDDP and found that seventeen were exceeding the maximum desirable radiation levels. In the New York area one radiologist was fired because his equipment repeatedly exceeded recommended levels.

The Guttman Institute uses equipment that much reduces the radiation reaching the skin or interior breast. The figure for Dr. Strax's equipment is $1/10$ rad (unit of absorbed radiation dose) per mammography exposure—similar to a chest X ray. "We have to unfrighten women about mammography and exams," Dr. Strax emphasizes.

A radiologist, Dr. Wende Logan, at Roswell Park Memorial Institute, Buffalo, New York, has demonstrated mammograms of good-quality resolution with $1/60$ rad reaching the center of the breast upon each view.

Any diagnostic tool will produce both false positives and false negatives. In 1977, Dr. Strax estimated that mammography and palpation each miss 20 percent of breast cancers. Use of all detection methods together, however, will miss only 5 to 10 percent. In Chapter 7, Pat states she owes her life to mammography which detected a malignancy missed in two physical exams. Irene (Chapter 16) had the opposite experience: mammography showed nothing definitive about her breast problem.

By late 1977 the BCDDP had located 2,500 previously unsuspected breast cancers. According to Dr. Arthur Holleb of ACS, 45 percent were found by mammography alone. The group age thirty-five to fifty accounted for about one-third (30 percent) of these malignancies, and 40 percent of their tumors were diagnosed by mammography alone.

Despite such figures, many physicians believe mammography for apparently asymptomatic women in this age group is wasteful, useless, and dangerous. Dr. Strax has called mammography "virtually of no value in women under fifty."

A *New York Times* editorial letter (10/8/77), referring to women in the Breast Cancer Demonstration Detection Projects who may have endured unnecessary mastectomy for tumors later judged benign, points out that "early detection of very small tumors, when they are difficult to diagnose as malignant or benign, is a double-edged sword."

The solution to this problem that affects the lives, hopes, and breasts of millions of women lies in better, safer diagnostic equipment and more agreement on how dangerous millimeter-sized breast cancers (or suspicious interphase cells) really are.

Xerography

Xerography (xeromammography), developed by the Xerox Corporation, is also an X-ray process. Images, which first appear on a specially charged plate or screen, are transferred to paper instead of film. The average radiation dosage it delivers to a woman's skin is lower than with direct-film mammography. The small bite-wing X-ray cardboards which a dentist inserts into your mouth are examples of the direct-film process.

The newest mammography units are CT (computerized tomography) machines. General Electric manufactures one type. This X-rays the breast in planes or cross-sections from many angles. Different kinds of tissue (fat, glands, skin, etc.) absorb rays at different rates. Data, recorded as numbers in a computer, are reconstructed as a picture on a screen, which can be photographed for a permanent visual record. This machine is similar to the CAT scanner which has proven to be especially useful for brain and abdominal X rays. A CT machine gives a more three-dimensional view of a tumor than is possible with conventional mammography equipment. Unfortunately, nowhere could I discover a machine used to ascertain the status of the underarm nodes. Ignorance about the condition of these nodes remains the rationale for many radical mastectomies.

Sonography—"X-ray-less X ray"

Mammography is effective and can be lifesaving to women at high risk for breast cancer. But because of the danger of accumulated radiation, another diagnostic tool is needed for regular screening of premenopausal or asymptomatic women. Ultrasound is one such tool, now used to supplement mammography.

Developed by the U.S. Navy to locate submarines and other submerged objects, it has already supplanted X ray in gynecology and obstetrics to obtain, for example, an image of an ovary or of a developing fetus without danger to mother or baby. Dr. Gilbert Baum, director of the ultrasound laboratory at Albert Einstein College of Medicine, Bronx, New York, is one researcher in the new field of ultrasound mammography.

High-frequency sound waves are projected onto the breast. Echoes bouncing off different kinds of tissues are converted by computerized equipment to images on a screen. The operator decides which images to color-photograph. Cancer appears as irregular patterns. To increase accuracy, two-dimensional motion studies using multiple sound beams or a single sweeping beam are now possible.

Part of the process resembles the "natural radar" by which bats bounce signals off the dark walls of caves to ascertain safe flight patterns.

Dr. Baum claims a 15 percent false negative rate. NCI is financing this ultrasound scanner research, with national distribution and testing expected about 1980.

Thermography

Because cancer attracts or creates its own blood vessels and supply, testing the breast for "hot spots"—areas of elevated temperature from increased circulation—is another diagnostic technique.

Memorial Sloan-Kettering Cancer Center is testing the accuracy of a process called GST (graphic stress telethermometry). A woman submerges her hands in cold water for fifteen minutes, sufficient to contract the blood vessels and cool the whole body, including the breasts. A malignant tumor, however, remains warmer when the heat sensor passes over the breast, and the equipment can also detect benign tumors. Data from the sensor goes to a computer that prints out a "numerical portrait" of the breast. An area of high score indicates a tumor.

Like sonography, this method complements X-ray mammography, but does not yet substitute for it.

Another heat device I learned of is BEBI (Breast Examination Bras, Inc.), developed by Dr. Eric Flam. This procedure is interesting because a woman can use it herself. In a doctor's office a woman is examined and fitted with a special bra. A machine photographs the normal thermal patterns in her breasts under the bra. Colored areas on the photos mark different temperatures in the patterns. She receives a set of photos to take with her.

Patterns in one breast will differ from the other, but patterns in the same breast should be consistent from month to month. The woman puts on the bra monthly and compares the patterns, which she sees reflected in a mirror, with the two photos she received in the doctor's office. The aim is to detect any sudden changes from her normal thermal patterns.

The system, designed to complement a woman's own monthly palpation of her breasts, consists of the bra, the photos, and a small illuminated mirror.

Dr. Flam's wife had breast cancer, a mastectomy, and cobalt therapy when she was under forty. She is a pharmacist and the mother of two children. When I asked, "How was the condition in your breast discovered?" she answered, "At home by my husband." This occurred before he developed the BEBI system. In 1977 he was demonstrating the bra at breast clinics.

He wrote me:

The BEBI bra itself is a thermograph. Clinical studies conducted by many investigators with about 100,000 patients have established the true positive rate of thermography to be about 85 percent. These studies span the years from 1966 to 1977 and are still going on. This rate compares favorably with a true positive rate of 85 percent for mammography (x-ray) and 82 percent for palpation. However, a very important finding in many of the studies is that changes in the thermal patterns and abnormal thermograms often occur from 6 months to 6 years *before* other indications of breast abnormality including cancers. This is so pronounced that an abnormal thermogram is regarded as a risk marker with many authorities feeling that a woman having this characteristic without any other clinical indication has a 9 to 15-fold greater risk of developing breast cancer than a woman with a normal thermogram.

I developed the BEBI system for a combination of technical and personal reasons. Technically, I knew that most breast cancers (95%) are first discovered by the women themselves, but too often at an advanced stage. I also knew that under controlled conditions, changes from the normal constant thermal patterns of a woman's breasts could be an early indication of changes in the breasts themselves. What I did was to successfully integrate these two factors to produce a safe breast self-examination system that could sense early changes in the breasts and alert the user to these changes so she could contact her doctor at *that* time. . . .

Many women now avoid exams and screening clinics because of the adverse publicity mammography has received. For them, any process, like the BEBI bra, that provides reliable views of breast contents without X ray is worth serious attention.

14 / *Elise*

Elise met me at the door of her apartment. It was a windblown night just before the holidays. I was glad to warm up over a drink, enjoying the art objects, including paintings and drawings of cats, she had collected.

One corner of her living room is devoted to electronic equipment. She earns her living as a singer, free-lance arranger, and copyist for musicians who play, but cannot read or notate, music. After hearing their work on tape, she notates or transcribes it, prior to its publication by a music company. She also reviews musical publications for a leading American magazine in the field.

A small woman with wavy auburn hair, Elise stressed the special crisis that mastectomy presents to the single woman, the woman undergoing menopause, the woman trying and needing to resume her former sexual life.

Due to events in her doctor's life, she also had to pursue part of her medical treatment on her own. She lacked the coordinated staging of physical and psychological care that someone like Dr. Thiessen (Chapter 15) offers his patients.

In December 1974, when Elise was fifty-six, she noticed something "not quite right" in her left breast. As she felt the area, she found a lump or swollen blood vessel toward the breastbone about an inch from the nipple.

Although she'd had a hysterectomy for fibroid tumors

when she was forty-two, that surgery had not removed her ovaries. Now she was having menopausal symptoms which her present doctor, a general practitioner she had consulted for many years, was treating with Premarin and a diuretic–weight reduction pill. "I had the courage to ask this doctor about the lump only because of Betty Ford. She made ladies aware of breast problems," Elise noted.

Although her doctor believed the lump was not serious, he advised her to observe it and made a mammography appointment for her at a clinic. The first date he could get was months away—May 1975. She describes him as "a kind man, a good doctor and diagnostician." In his mid-sixties, he was on the eve of planned retirement. He advised Elise that he would be unavailable for further care or consultation, and gave her names of another general practitioner and a surgeon (gynecologist).

While she waited for mammography, she "felt the lump getting harder. It was dimpling the skin. I realized I must get the courage to do something about this. I'd have to ask questions of somebody. I called the new GP to ask for more diuretic pills because I was gaining weight." During this visit, which occurred in March 1975, she asked, "While I'm here, will you look at this lump?"

After examining it, the doctor stated, "If you were my sister, I would tell you not to wait, to go see about it immediately." He got her a mammography appointment. When the radiology staff handed her the large envelope of X-ray prints to carry to her doctor, she thought it "a big nuisance because cancer couldn't happen to me. You don't get cancer—other people get cancer."

When this doctor examined the mammograms, he said, "You should consult a surgeon."

However, the surgeon recommended by her original doctor proved to be out of town. Her new general practitioner got her a consultation with another surgeon for the following day. "When an emergency presented itself, the doctors were concerned—and these were strangers," she noted. Of the surgeon who, of course, recommended biopsy with mastectomy, if needed, she asked, "What will I do?" He answered, "You can wear a falsie." This merely intensified the shock she was feeling. "The world without a breast had never existed for me."

Because the hospital could not admit her immediately, the surgeon instructed her to pack a bag and be on call each day from nine to four, should a vacancy occur. This period was trying. "I went through ten days of knowing I needed an operation, wondering whether they would call, being relieved each day when they hadn't." A call to the American Cancer Society for help in getting a hospital room did not succeed. ACS' major purposes are education, research, and a certain amount of community service, such as cancer detection programs.

Finally Elise decided, "This is crazy," and phoned the surgeon's secretary, asking, "If I wanted a private room instead of semiprivate, could I go?" The secretary easily booked her into a private room at another hospital.

Private rooms earn more money for a hospital, but that is not the total problem. Often, while I was doing this book, the thought crossed my mind that cancer, including breast cancer, affected men also. How many men would tolerate such delays and problems in treatment or the fact that easing a patient's emotions during such crises seems of such minor interest that no one apparently counted whether it was ten—or fifty—days Elise had to wait? The fact that one patient is just that—one patient—and busy medical professionals must deal with x^2 numbers of them is supposed to justify everything. If a patient dares complain, she is apt to be silenced with a rejoinder like, "Well, it didn't kill you, did it?"—a minimalist response reminiscent of frontier America or the hills of Puritan New England.

When I asked whether anything comforting or useful that someone did lingered in Elise's mind, she replied, "*I* did something. I'm not a religious person, but the day of my hospital entry, I tried to get into a synagogue. When it was locked, I went to a Greek Orthodox church." There she prayed for "the strength to withstand whatever happened. I didn't pray not to have a mastectomy." In Freudian terms, Elise's subconscious inner wisdom was preparing her for what she couldn't yet accept consciously.

She also remembered addressing her breast: "You betrayed me."

At the hospital she signed the consent form for a simultaneous biopsy/mastectomy. "I was terrified of the operation. I wanted it over with. I wanted it once and for all. I was not capable of listening to a verdict and acting on it later. I wanted it all over with so I could get back to living."

The next thing she recalled was regaining consciousness. "When I came to, I sensed the breast was taken off. I felt the bandages and drain." When her arm swelled, she realized the lymph nodes were gone.

She requested a Reach to Recovery volunteer (Chapter 23). Whether through accident or planning, the wife of a friend in the music world came to visit. This woman, about forty years old, also a mastectomee, was wearing a black turtleneck sweater, which she removed along with her blouse. Elise saw—one breast. "I still didn't connect that with mastectomy. Older women with pendulous breasts had cancer, not me. I wouldn't look at myself. I kept my eyes closed when the nurses washed me. I knew I had no breast, but I wouldn't look at it."

Of her April 1975 modified radical surgery, eight-day hospital stay, and agonizing prior arrangements, she remarked, "Within the boundary of what was available to me, I got good care."

She remembered going home. "I called my roommate and asked for three or four bras, and stockings to stuff into whichever one might fit the best."

In the hospital Elise's surgeon told her that some follow-up therapy would be necessary, and he recommended either irradiation or chemotherapy. She again called the American Cancer Society, this time for further information on chemotherapy, and was unable to obtain any literature. Finally a friend in one of her classes introduced her to a general practitioner, who consulted with Elise's surgeon. She would receive irradiation "as a preventive measure."

She underwent the standard course of twenty-five irradiation treatments over a period of weeks. She recalled especially the superbly functioning radiotherapy team at the hospital where she was treated. "These people made me feel euphoric. . . . The radiation experience is strange. You're alone in the room. The machinery is like something from Mount Palomar. The machine focuses. You are the center of the universe." Bone and liver scans, which she also received, "gave me a claustrophobic feeling." The vast machine that is used passes close down on the body.

"I was afraid of being nauseous but wasn't at all. I did have trouble swallowing after treatments. I was determined not to be incapacitated." During radiotherapy she did lose some weight and "was glad."

Problems, physical and emotional, awaited her, however. "I haven't worked through my feelings of anger, of 'Why me?' yet. I remember crying in anger and frustration. I went to a bra shop and felt so ugly." She discovered she was walking lopsided, hunched over from the absence of weight in the missing breast. She had to retrain herself how to move. "I can walk without a prosthesis now. I can look at myself in the mirror now—one more second every day. I had to force myself to look at myself."

Win Ann Winkler, author of an excellent book called *Post-Mastectomy,* details a few of her emotions, similar to Elise's:

. . . the rosy pictures people painted for me as to how well I was doing only increased my sense of outrage. Logic told me that I had taken the only sensible course of action open to me by seeking competent help when I did, and it was easier having the experience behind me than ahead. But the infuriating, "Why did this have to happen to *me?*" seemed to blot out any rational thoughts I had been able to muster. On top of that, I had the feeling that something had been put over on me—that the decision was taken out of my hands. True, I had signed for the mastectomy when I signed for the biopsy. . . .

. . . there came a day when, looking in the mirror, I decided to stop looking at the scar and start looking at the way my body moved. For me, one positive outcome of my mastectomy was that I became aware of inner grace rather than geometric surfaces.

However, before this point she had to endure many more moments when she felt, "One more pep talk and I'll scream!"

Shortly before our interview, Elise had joined a weekly postmastectomy counseling group that was discussing how to cope with stress. Although she found it helpful, the predominance of married women and those needing to discuss the physical side effects of chemotherapy sometimes made it difficult. The focus on stress intrigued her because she had experienced much tension at the time of her father's death shortly before her breast lump appeared.

Elise had an unusually late menopause, ending only four months before our interview when she was fifty-nine. She reported "five years of menopausal symptoms" that increased her physical discomfort and retarded her adjustment to the mastectomy.

Finally she discussed her sexual feelings. "I was helped by the literature I read, except that none of the books deals frankly with sexual problems. These people say things like, 'The right answer will come to you' or 'You're the same wonderful person you were before' or 'If anyone can't face your mastectomy, then this is the wrong relationship for you.'

"Because I grew up in the era of the Lana Turner sweater girl, I felt I had lost a certain part of my attractiveness. I'm not attractive to *me* now."

As with other mastectomees, the problem is as much physical as psychological. Because of cut nerves and scar tissue, nearly three years after surgery her breast area is perceived as a combination of deadness and oversensitivity. "It is nerve-wracking to be touched. I had a strong sex drive, but mastectomy destroyed any sex feeling I have. It's inhibiting and distressing now to make love without a bra on. It has made sexual experiences painful and unrewarding." Although a new lover has told her that her lack of a breast doesn't matter, "equally important is what I think of myself. I'm not yet capable of relating in a sexual way. And I used to be proud of my figure. My breasts were a source of sexual stimulation."

Both married and single women of all ages share the fear that a mastectomy may end the enjoyment of sexual life by introducing self-consciousness or destroying sensation. A forty-five-year-old married woman wrote her feelings to her Boston surgeon, Dr. Oliver Cope. Her husband tells me that the fact I have only one breast makes no difference to him, that he is grateful to have me around, alive and well—and I believe him. But in our intimate moments, it is a hard thing for me to do to present him with this disfigurement. One breast by itself is rather obscene, I think. My husband says it doesn't look that way to him, but it looks that way to me.

I can truthfully say that the loss of a breast has not affected our lovemaking to any extent.

I've just realized that I have told a lie, but didn't recognize it until I saw it set down on paper. Our lovemaking as far as tenderness and wanting one another has not been affected, but my enjoyment of it has, because my left breast was always extremely sensitive and was one of my most important erogenous zones. Now it isn't there anymore, and I miss it to this day.

There is no immediate answer for such problems. Clichés ("You can resume anytime, dear," "You're the same wonderful woman you always were") merely increase indignation. Such statements reassure some people but infuriate others. This is another area where surgeons might demonstrate more courage by spending a few minutes inquiring into a woman's life-style while they explain the possible side effects of mastectomy. And women, too, need to demonstrate more honesty in mentioning their sexual lives when mastectomy is discussed. One solution may be to choose a doctor whose attitude toward women is compassionate and modern.

Since some form of lumpectomy plus irradiation or chemotherapy now seems as effective (Chapter 15) as mastectomy in controlling minimal breast cancer, a woman like Elise, to whom a breast means physical and sexual attractiveness, should have been offered this alternative. Not every woman will want it. Some, like Rita or Pat, prefer the security that radical mastectomy seems to give. But *it is cruel not to offer the lesser operation,* especially to an older woman, whenever a doctor suspects, or she states, that life without a breast would be unimaginable. Even if the breast must be removed later, she will know that her particular doctor "was not a mad cutter," that he did what he could to save the breast initially.

Some doctors fear that women will sue them for malpractice if they fail to perform a radical mastectomy—the hallowed and still current treatment for breast cancer. One solution would be a revised consent form that, besides allowing medical personnel to perform all the usual duties related to surgery, would state that the woman has been informed of various possible procedures and treatments relevant to her case and that, based on the results of biopsy, she agrees to a lesser surgery under certain conditions and radical mastectomy under other conditions (size, kind, and position of tumor, lymph node involvement, etc.). Veronica Gardos (Chapter 18) informally negotiated such an agreement. Even with surgeons who still demand the one-stage operation (biopsy combined with mastectomy), a woman would at least feel before and afterward that options had been discussed with her, whether or not they applied in her case.

Elise's latest problem, also mastectomy-related, is renewed swelling of her arm. Her surgeon has recommended that she wear an elastic sleeve.

Despite her anger at the facts of cancer and her disfigurement, Elise has experienced moments of relative peace. Psychiatrists and women themselves speculate on which kind or age of patient bears the stress of illness best. Elise decided, "I thought because of my age I was better able to cope than a young woman. Better it should happen to me than a younger person, I thought." After surgery, various friends proved supportive. They "pulled me through. I was not allowed to brood."

And she retains her particular verve. After all our talk of problems, she reminded me with a laugh, "Remember I function more than 100 percent with clothes on!"

15 / Saving Breast and Life: New Treatment Methods

It has been calculated that there are perhaps fourteen different combinations possible for the woman with breast cancer. Opinions differ widely among the experts in this country as well as abroad. Treatments vary all the way from a needle diagnosis followed by radiation therapy to supraradical surgery and the many combinations in between. . . . When we add such procedures as oophorectomy, chemotherapy, and radiation therapy before or after surgery, the possible combinations are literally legion.

—DR. PHILIP STRAX, *Early Detection*

No topic related to breast cancer has aroused more recent controversy than treatment methods. Reasons for this lie in

• The enigma of cancer itself.
• The variability of breast cancer in particular that requires at least a five-year follow-up to determine research results. Perfectionists insist on ten- to twenty-year data for either prospective or retrospective studies.
• The fact that physicians espousing the century-old radical mastectomy do not easily accept alternate therapies, even when these appear equally effective.

The five-year survival rate after radical mastectomy for disease apparently localized to the breast is an impressive

80 to 85 percent. This is a general average achieved by surgeons throughout the United States; some will achieve more, some less. Following and qualifying this, however, are innumerable sets of treatment data that can be explained more by the nature of the disease than by any lack of surgical skill.

The five-year survival rate for metastasized breast cancer is about 60 percent. The ten-year rate drops to 45 percent. Both of these statistics refer to women who underwent some form of radical mastectomy. And here is a sentence from Herbert Seidman of the American Cancer Society, by no means a group advocating alternate therapies: "At the point in their development at which breast cancers become clinically detectable, it is clear that the behavior of tumors ranges from those that will kill quickly, whatever is done, to those that will progress slowly, whether or not anything is done."

In other words, *no one kind of breast surgery alone saves lives automatically.* Much depends upon tumor type and location, the surgeon's skill, the stage of the disease, and the success of follow-up (adjuvant) therapy in combating wandering cancer cells even in women whose underarm nodes appeared "clean."

To be fair, I should also mention that the overall five-year survival rate for totally untreated breast cancer (rarely seen in the United States today) is only 20 percent; the ten-year rate is less than 5 percent. In fact, it approaches zero (data from 1926 to 1962).

The poor, including black women, tend to have their breast cancer diagnosed at a later stage. NCI data from the early seventies shows that in nearly half (48 percent) of white women diagnosed as having the disease, the cancer was localized to the breast, while it was localized in only 33 percent of black women. In two out of three black women diagnosed as having breast cancer, it had already spread to the nodes or beyond. This is tragic because black women get *less* breast cancer than white women of northern European ancestry in the first place.

The two points to stress are: (1) radical mastectomy with or without further therapy will not cure all breast cancer patients; and (2) partial mastectomy, also called "lumpectomy," with follow-up treatment is now curing just as many, according to recent and long-term research.

Partial mastectomy has various names, depending on how much tissue is removed. Strictly speaking, *lumpectomy* removes only the lump in an excisional biopsy procedure. Partial mastectomy, also called *wedge* or *segmental resection,* removes a larger tissue portion—flat, oval, or triangular in shape, depending on the pattern of tumor spread—along with or beneath the skin. The final scar may be nearly invisible if the surgeon can, or chooses to, pierce the dark area (areola) near the nipple, using that entrance to reach and remove tumor-containing tissues. Closing stitches (sutures) are fine nylon thread, painless to snip out a few days later after the adhesive bandages come off. If the removed area is small enough, the breast resumes its former shape. All these partial procedures aim to remove the tumor safely while preserving the remaining breast tissue, nipple, and skin.

What all this means is that no woman any longer need be ordered or intimidated into a radical mastectomy by a surgeon who sneers or shouts that without it, she'll be dead in five years or that if keeping her breast matters to her, she must be a prostitute or nymphomaniac.

However, if radical mastectomy, done by a surgeon that a woman likes and trusts, *is* the choice that will give or has given her peace of mind, it is not by any means the wrong choice—for her. The era of sure cancer cure and prevention—beyond cancer treatment—honestly does not exist yet.

I merely believe many *more* women should be able to state of their surgeons, "I felt he wouldn't do more than he had to, that he wasn't a mad cutter. I trusted what he said, and felt he wouldn't lie to me about my life."

If you feel at high risk for breast cancer or if you face the need to choose a physician for surgery or more routine breast care, here is what you should know to choose wisely.

Background: The Halsted Radical

First of all, it is past time to dethrone the radical mastectomy, developed in the United States about 1880 by Dr. William Stewart Halsted, as the automatic treatment of choice for every woman's breast cancer. Halsted's ten-year survival rate was also about 50 percent of his patients. Because many arrived with ulcerated, orange-sized tumors that filled one whole breast, the surgeries he performed were aggressive—the *standard radical* (which removes breast, underarm nodes, chest muscles) and the *extended* or *supraradical* (which adds rib sections to get at the internal mammary nodes near the breastbone, and which may also excise nodes above the collarbone).

It may surprise you that by today's standards, *none* of Halsted's patients with such grave signs of metastasized disease as skin ulceration or palpable lymph nodes would be considered "operable" or would receive mastectomy at all. The reason is that irradiation and chemotherapy now exist as supplements or alternates to surgery. Halsted had only surgery, which he perfected from techniques pioneered in Germany. He is no ignorant villain to be scorned; he experimented with equipment and medical procedures later used throughout the United States, such as certain suturing techniques, rubber gloves, sterile dressings, cocaine as anesthesia. Before him, for example, 10 percent of the women receiving a simple mastectomy (removal of only the breast) died of the surgery itself—from hemorrhage or infection.

His errors stemmed from inadequate knowledge of the disease itself—its initial methods of spread, and its apparently latent period after original surgery.

A general surgeon, Halsted based his major work with breast cancer on just 133 cases, only 75 of which he followed more than three years. His first scientific paper on breast cancer was titled, "The Results of Operation for the Cure of Cancer of the Breast Performed at the Johns Hopkins Hospital from June, 1889, to January, 1894." He dared use the word "cure" because, by modern standards, his criteria were minimal: women free of local recurrence for one year after surgery had "hope of a cure"; women free for three years were considered a definite cure. Unfortunately only six of his first group of fifty lived more than three years, although any prolonged survival was considered remarkable at the time. What he never grasped was that breast cancer can seed itself via the bloodstream as well as the lymph nodes. His impassioned surgical war against nodes, therefore, could never, and never will, succeed in all cases—not in 1890, and not in 1990.

In an article on breast cancer history, Dr. Kenneth J. Meyer comments: "In devising his operation Halsted sought a method to prevent local recurrence of cancer of the breast and considered freedom from skin recurrence cure of breast cancer. He did not even discuss survival until his second paper in 1898. Death from internal metastasis was not the surgeon's responsibility."

Like his surgery, Halsted's logic was flawless: no breast . . . no breast skin . . . no breast cancer—and a stunning example of the cliché: "The operation was a success, but the patient died."

By 1907, when he had accumulated experience and records from 232 patients, he realized that a five-year follow-up was necessary. The women themselves, in life and in death, refuted his finest efforts.

I have dwelt on Dr. Halsted's simultaneous success/failure because the reasons for it—ignorance, arrogance, overspecialization—have continued to plague U.S. cancer research and treatment, especially when these touch an organ like the breast whose value to a woman is something only a rare surgeon wants to admit or confront.

As part of the U.S. Senate (94th Congress) Subcommittee Hearings on Breast Cancer during 1976, Dr. Vincent DeVita, director of NCI's Division of Cancer Treatment, wrote:

Halsted did not develop his procedure for patients with small primary tumors with no palpable lymph glands. He, and surgeons before him, rarely saw such patients, since early diagnosis was veritably unheard of. Surely, Halsted would have questioned whether a radical procedure was necessary for such patients. Certainly, surgeons in this country should have questioned it a long time ago. . . .

In patients without lymph gland involvement, it is very questionable as to whether a radical procedure is indicated because the disease *has not* spread to the axilla [armpit]; in those with axillary gland involvement by itself, radical mastectomy is both too much and not enough. . . . We continue to recommend mastectomy . . . in many cases because of the *need to know the status of lymph glands in the axilla* in regard to further decisions about postoperative treatment with drugs. We have no other reliable tests to determine their status at the present time.

One of the reasons for lack of enthusiasm in studying less radical approaches for the control of local breast cancer is that they were, and are, unlikely to produce *better survival* results than radical mastectomy, just, at best, equivalent survival with less morbidity.

To translate this from "medicalese," what he's saying is that women who receive lesser procedures can live just as long and in better general health and appearance, therefore probably in better mental health, than those who receive more drastic procedures.

Dr. George Crile, author of *What Every Woman Should Know About the Breast Cancer Controversy,* also testified at these hearings. Even he, despite years of being slandered as the flaming radical of lumpectomy, does the lesser operation only "if the tumor is small and peripheral and the breast is ample." Medicine is by and large so conservative a profession that any practitioner who deviates the slightest from practices long based on precedent is considered suspect, even when this might benefit the patient. Obvious deviations involved in malpractice, however, are often hidden or ignored by the same doctors.

Of 91,000 breast cancer patients diagnosed yearly, how many continue to receive some form of radical mastectomy?

When I telephoned the National Center for Health Statistics, a librarian gave me the latest figures available from an NCI volume called *Cancer Patient Survival,* covering data for the early seventies. The breakdown is shown in Figure 10.

A little arithmetic shows that fully 92 percent of the patients received surgery. Figures for the late seventies would not differ substantially, except that the use of chemotherapy and irradiation as adjuncts to surgery has increased. Lumpectomy alone may account for some of this surgery, but it is likely that the majority of that 92 percent received—and continue to receive—radical mastectomy.

Recent research has involved testing the results of "combined modalities" (lesser surgeries with and without chemotherapy or irradiation). Because of the nature of breast

Figure 10. DIFFERENT KINDS OF TREATMENT
RECEIVED BY U.S. BREAST CANCER PATIENTS

KIND OF TREATMENT	PERCENT OF PATIENTS
Surgery only	57
Surgery + irradiation	30
Surgery + chemotherapy	2
Surgery, irradiation, chemotherapy	3
Irradiation only	2
Chemotherapy only	2
Irradiation + chemotherapy	2
No treatment	2
	100

End Results Section, NCI, Cancer Patient Survival, 1950–1973. Data
from 100 U.S. hospitals.

cancer, remember that any research result—no matter how
spectacular—can be attacked as "provisional," "inconclusive,"
or some other condemnatory adjective, if one chooses.

Basing their findings upon the results of a combination of simple mastectomy and irradiation as done in Scotland
during World War II (when surgeons with enough training to
perform the radical mastectomy were caring for soldiers), Dr.
M. V. Peters in Toronto and Dr. S. Mustakallio in Finland
have published the survival rates of different forms of lumpectomy (partial mastectomy), followed by radiotherapy to
breast and underarm nodes. One of Dr. Peters' articles, based
on eighty patients, is "Wedge Resection and Irradiation: An
Effective Treatment of Early Breast Cancer" (*Journal of the
American Medical Society* 200:144, 1967).

One of Dr. Mustakallio's articles is "Conservative
Treatment of Breast Cancer—Review of 25 Years Followup"
(*Clinical Radiology* 23:110–16, 1972). Summarizing work with
702 patients, this report gives a five-year survival rate of 80
percent, a ten-year rate of 60 percent, and a fifteen-year rate
of 47 percent.

Even the radicals of radical mastectomy must confront
their own long-term survival figure that hovers around 45
percent—or less. In "Longterm Followup of Breast Cancer
Patients: The 30-Year Report" (*Cancer* 33:1145–50, 4/74), Drs.
Frank Adair and Guy Robbins, both of Breast Service, De-

partment of Surgery, Memorial Hospital, New York, reported on 1,458 patients with "potentially curable invasive clinical breast cancer" given radical mastectomy between 1940 and 1943. About 60 percent—836 women—eventually died of cancer. The rate for survivors at thirty years postmastectomy amounted to just 38 percent. Of course, in the forties before chemotherapy, a systemic attack on cancer did not exist.

Chemotherapy and Irradiation

In 1957 the National Surgical Adjuvant Breast Project (NSABP) was organized in the United States to evaluate various treatment methods. Coordinated by Dr. Bernard Fisher of the University of Pittsburgh, it now receives data from more than fifty institutions, including several hundred surgeons, radiologists, oncologists, and pathologists. In 1958 it began clinical trials on the first drug, Thio TEPA, that seemed useful against breast cancer. It was employed chiefly as an adjuvant to radical mastectomy. In 1972, NSABP added trials with L-PAM (L-phenylalanine mustard, a descendant of the World War I chemical warfare compounds out of which chemotherapy evolved). In 1975, trials with 5-FU (5-fluorouracil) began.

In general, chemotherapy is most successful against small tumors after the main tumor mass has been surgically removed. Drugs such as L-PAM are also more effective in premenopausal women, probably because they block body production or use of estrogen as well as killing cancer cells. They effect a temporary, chemical oophorectomy (surgical removal of the ovaries). Seventy-five percent of premenopausal women cease menstruating while receiving chemotherapy, for instance.

To quote just one sentence from a 1977 report to the ACS by Dr. David Rose, Wisconsin Clinical Cancer Center, Madison: "Overall, the likelihood of remaining tumor-free is significantly greater for the patients given CMF [a three-drug combination] compared with those treated by mastectomy alone."

Tamoxifen, developed in Britain, is effective against postmenopausal breast cancer in women whose tumors are estrogen-dependent. It is now in limited use in the United States at the University of Minnesota and at Southwestern Medical School, University of Texas, among other locations.

In 1977, Dr. Fisher stated, "There is no question that chemotherapy for breast cancer is here to stay. Now it's a matter of finding out what chemotherapy is best for which patients. Using chemotherapy, I have every reason to believe that in the immediate future lesser surgery will be as effective as radical mastectomy in treating breast cancer."

It is estimated that by the time a breast cancer is discovered, tumor stem cells have already spread beyond the underarm lymph nodes in 50 percent of the patients—beyond treatment by either irradiation or mastectomy—and regardless also of whether these nodes *"look* clean." In 1976 Dr. Fisher's "Ten-Year Followup Results of Patients in a Cooperative Clinical Trial Evaluating Surgical Adjuvant Chemotherapy" reported among many other data that 25 percent of the patients with apparently negative nodes (and 75 percent of the patients with positive nodes) "displayed a treatment failure by ten years." This suggests that some form of chemotherapy should be given to many more women with cancer at all stages, including minimal or localized cancer.

However, chemotherapy, like irradiation, not only kills cancer cells but can cause new tumors in some patients, probably by weakening the body's immunodefense system. An estimate is that 5 percent to 10 percent of chemotherapy patients will get a second or third primary cancer (a tumor in a new location unrelated to the original cancer). Chemotherapists defend themselves by saying that such a risk is minimal compared to the risks associated with the primary tumor and that patients are at least *living* long enough to assess the subsequent risks.

One research study, from 1971 through 1974, compared radical mastectomy to simple mastectomy, with and without postoperative irradiation. In 1976 Dr. Fisher reported to Congress "no significant difference in results between treatment groups."

In 1976, Dr. Fisher's project obtained approval to begin comparing the results of a modified radical mastectomy for stage I (minimal) breast cancer with two other approaches:

(1) partial mastectomy + axillary node dissection (Veronica's surgery—see chapter 18); and (2) partial mastectomy + node dissection + irradiation.

Coordinating Individual Care

To gain direct information on current methods of treating breast diseases, especially cancer, from a surgeon's viewpoint, I questioned Dr. Eugene Thiessen of Strang Clinic-Preventive Medicine Institute, Manhattan, where he is chief of the Breast Disease Clinic. He is also on the staff of New York University Medical Center.

Dr. Thiessen is a general surgeon who has specialized in breast diseases and the array of treatment—various surgeries, chemotherapy, psychological counseling—that a woman afflicted with breast cancer may need at different stages.

His aim is to avoid the frightening fragmentation of care that can happen when a woman finds herself shuttling from internist or gynecologist to surgeon, back to internist, maybe on to a radiotherapist or oncologist. "Each does his little thing, and the average general surgeon may do as few as two mastectomies per year," Dr. Thiessen observed. None takes overall responsibility or concern for her, and none is trained or apt to offer help with the psychological effects of disease and treatment. It is also possible (see Elise, Chapter 14) that for some reason she doesn't get a clear recommendation about treatment from the first doctor she consults and must proceed on her own.

"I take responsibility for any of the decisions about a woman's care," Dr. Thiessen emphasized. If hormonal manipulation in a premenopausal woman is indicated for an estrogen-dependent tumor, he will do an oophorectomy (removal of the ovaries).

I was particularly curious about Dr. Thiessen's positions on standard radical mastectomy, radiotherapy, and "lumpectomy" (although the amount of tissue removed usually exceeds the lump). I also wondered how he treats benign disease.

"I haven't done the standard Halsted radical mastectomy for ten years," Dr. Thiessen began. "I do a modified radical if any kind of radical seems indicated for a particular patient." If a woman comes to him with a lump that appears malignant, he orders a work-up that includes mammography, chest X ray, enzyme and blood studies, and total body scanning. "If all evidence indicates the cancer is limited to the breast, I recommend that all breast tissue be removed. If after complete evaluation, I learn the cancer has already spread beyond the breast, I do no mastectomy but recommend biopsy of the breast and any other tumor, followed by radiation."

Having an overall view of the patient, he can more easily heed a woman's competing health problems. He mentioned a patient, approximately sixty years old, whose breast cancer had not only metastasized to the spine but who had nephritis, an infection that caused an abscessed, nonfunctional kidney. "If I put her on immunosuppressant drugs, this would kill her because the drugs would allow the nephritis to spread without hindrance." Because chemotherapy attacks all rapidly dividing body cells, including lymphocytes that help fight infection, it can temporarily lower a woman's resistance.

Besides lumpectomy for advanced disease, he will also recommend this surgery for a small malignant lump in an older woman, followed by radiation, when the disease is confined to the breast.

"How old is older?" I immediately asked.

"The answer depends on evaluating her total situation and history. If this is her first breast lump at age fifty-eight, her chance of malignancy is high. If it's her first breast lump at twenty-two or she's a young woman with history of benign lumps, there's a much lower chance."

We discussed Dr. George Crile's views on lumpectomy. "I have great respect for Dr. Crile, but I don't agree with his data, his animal research. His human data are based on insufficient numbers of women. I feel his data are insufficient to say lumpectomy, plus X form of treatment, is sufficient against breast cancer.

"You know his primary treatment remains radical mastectomy. In other cases, he will do lumpectomy if a woman won't accept any other form of treatment. I feel his criteria evaluating a tumor suitable for lumpectomy are vague. It should not be 'too big,' 'too near the nipple.' Well, any lump in the upper half of the breast, compared with the lower half, will be 'near the nipple.'

"However, Dr. Crile has caused people to rethink their automatic acceptance of radical mastectomy as the standard form of treatment for every breast cancer. You know, before and after Halsted, there were attempts to do lesser surgeries. Radical mastectomy really rose to prominence in the thirties in this country."

For a younger woman Dr. Thiessen does a modified radical because of his views on the danger of accumulated radiation from radiotherapy, should she have it following a lumpectomy. "I became aware of the inconsistency in professionals' attitude toward use of radiation. On the one hand, NCI is so concerned about danger of routine mammography in young women that they recommend it only for women over fifty now. On the other hand, surgeons are treating young women's breast cancer with radiation. Some are giving 3,000 to 5,000 rads total during a radiation series following lumpectomy. How do they know such doses won't cause as many tumors as they prevent over her life span?

"In a young woman who has lumpectomy, the linings of the duct system, the cells from which breast cancer commonly arises, are still intact. You may have eliminated one focus of cancer with this radiation, but breast cancer is multicentric. Minimal *in situ* cancers may recur in other spots in that breast.

"Radiotherapists may be contributing to new cancer. They can't give a guarantee it won't recur, and nobody is telling the patient that the amounts of radiation given can cause new cancers in some breasts. For example, young people with Hodgkin's disease, irradiated for a first tumor, are more apt to develop a second tumor in the area of radiation than those not irradiated."

This is one reason why some physicians are using chemotherapy following surgery for women with nodal involvement. Dr. Thiessen uses multiple different drugs, including CMF (cyclophosphamide, methotrexate, fluorouracil), much researched in Italy by a team headed by Dr. Gianni Bonadonna. Dr. Thiessen had two comments. "Remember that Bonadonna was not using it alone to achieve success against breast cancer. All his patients have radical or modified radical surgery. No patient had a lesser surgery." He admitted, "Chemotherapy is a shot in the dark. And we have no end point for how to measure or prescribe it." Since its success is based on what does *not* happen, recurrence or metastasis, "there's no way to prove—nor can you tell a patient—that her recurrence at five years would have come at three without chemotherapy or might not have come at all."

Dr. Thiessen does not consider benign disease a prelude to, or even a risk factor for, breast cancer. "Benign disease is a wastepaper basket diagnosis. It is so common it means nothing. Autopsy studies have shown change associated with benign disease in 70 percent to 75 percent of women dying of all causes. If a doctor removes a benign lump, he is implying that benign lumps become cancerous. I don't believe this."

Nor does he aspirate (drain) fluid-filled cysts because thickening of cells in an abnormal area may return. Then biopsy may be needed anyway. He does take a patient's history. Again, the most likely lump for biopsy, rather than watching, is a first lump in an older woman.

Dr. Thiessen is one of the few surgeons I found who take a genuine interest in his patients' psychological rehabilitation to the point of starting and continuing participation in a counseling group (S.H.A.R.E) at the Strang Clinic. Other similar groups have since formed. A trained counselor and a medical social worker assist. Women discuss the emotional problems uniquely related to breast cancer. "This is a rap session, not psychotherapy," he noted. "It certainly has met a need, and it has helped me develop and understand patients and help them feel they're not alone. I meet regularly with the group." The discussions cover clothing, job discrimination, and attitudes about physical, sexual, and family matters because "breast cancer is a family disease." A woman needs to help her family understand—and to be helped by them.

Like much group therapy, it is private and special-purpose—limited to postmastectomy patients.

Treatment without Mastectomy

For another view of combined treatments—minus *any* form of radical mastectomy—I quote from Dr. Oliver Cope, a surgeon at Massachusetts General Hospital, Boston, and Professor of Surgery at Harvard Medical School. Dr. Cope has not performed mastectomy of any kind since 1960 although he did it routinely for thirty years until he met his first two patients who refused it. It was these women themselves who used the only power that remained to them—the ability to say no *effectively*—that changed both his mind and his methods. He also noticed that patients with supposedly good prognoses died eventually of cancer—despite his finest surgery.

In his book, *The Breast: Its Problems—Benign and Malignant—and How to Deal with Them,* he describes what happened:

I am just old enough to have seen patients with advanced neglected cancer of the breast. . . . As an intern and resident, from 1928 through 1932, I was schooled in the performance of a radical mastectomy by two of Boston's foremost surgeons, Drs. E. P. Richardson and E. D. Churchill. . . . I concentrated on the techniques needed to become an expert. I accepted the traditional thinking and asked no questions.

Despite three particular women in 1943, through whom he was "brought up short by the mutilation and cruelty of losing a breast suffered by each of those patients," he continued radical mastectomies until 1956.

Then, for the first time, I met a patient who refused to have a mastectomy. It was not that she was afraid of an operation—she had asked me to operate on her goiter—but she was adamant about her breast, and I had to arrange an alternative for her.

He performed a lumpectomy, followed by irradiation.

Then, in 1958, the widow of one of my teachers of medicine refused to have a mastectomy in any form, and told my why. She made me look at the cruelty of my trade, the surgeon's trade. . . . It was she who forced me finally to look critically at the operation of radical mastectomy to see just what it was accomplishing. I had to ask myself three questions. Was I justified in acquiescing to her demand to provide her with a less mutilating treatment? Had I harmed the earlier patient? And should I have found a way to convince both patients to accept the mastectomy? There was now no escape; I had to examine what radical mastectomy really amounts to. As I looked, the evidence against the operation was convincing; so convincing indeed that I did my last radical mastectomy in 1960.

Simultaneously he also investigated emotional aspects of breast cancer. He is honest enough to admit, "I have never known a woman who did not profoundly resent the loss of her breast," however stoic she may *appear* as she begs fate to accept her breast in trade for her life.

Dr. Cope uses the Ackerman system of tumor classification (L. V. Ackerman and J. Rosai, "The Pathology of Tumors, Part Four: Grading, Staging, and Classification of Neoplasms," *CA: A Cancer Journal for Clinicians* 21:368, 1971). His recommended treatment regime involves:

Type I, carcinoma *in situ*, noninvasive, 5% to 10% of breast cancer. Treatment: excision of tumor [lumpectomy].

Type II, slightly invasive of surrounding tissue and rest of breast, 10% to 15 % of breast cancer. Treatment: excision, followed by irradiation only of breast.

Type III, spread to lymph nodes and throughout breast, 35% to 45%. Treatment: excision; irradiation of both breast and nodes; chemotherapy "promptly and for long periods."

Type IV, spread by blood vessels to several breast areas, to chest wall, skin, 35% to 45%. Treatment: excision; irradiation of breast and nodes; chemotherapy.

Types III and IV involve five to seven weeks of radiotherapy—"a full tumor dose, not a lesser adjuvant dose"—followed by about two years of chemotherapy. In certain cases, Dr. Cope excises some underarm lymph nodes for examination in addition to the primary tumor.

Two years of chemotherapy are bearable, of course, only when, as with Irene (Chapter 16), dosages and drugs are carefully monitored to reduce side effects. The results of Dr.

Cope's work with 180 patients are described in a journal article, "Limited Surgical Excision as the Basis of a Comprehensive Therapy for Cancer of the Breast" (*American Journal of Surgery* 131:400–7, 1976).

A further aspect of his treatment is his refusal to rely on results of frozen sections, performed on the tumor by the pathologist while the patient lies anesthetized. What he terms "blood vessel invasion" by the tumor type IV is a serious indication that cancer cells have already begun to wander the body. Such invasion

cannot be excluded by the pathologist during the operation by so-called frozen section. The freezing of such tissue and the subsequent slicing of the icy tissue inevitably distort the patterns of the cells, and the fine points such as blood vessel invasion are rarely discernible. It takes two to three days of special staining and study to be sure of this finding, but where it exists there is no point in subjecting the patient to a radical operation or, indeed, any form of mastectomy.

Irradiation by Implantation

Finally I want to describe radioactive implants for breast cancer. The formal name is "interstitial radiation therapy." It involves embedding tiny bits of short-lived radioactive isotopes in and around malignant tissue. For three to five days the patient carries within her breast thin, flexible plastic tubes bearing "seeds" of iridium 192. The number of tubes inserted depends on the size of the tumor. For small tumors (no more than 4 centimeters—1½ inches), implantation follows lumpectomy. Larger tumors, left in place, actually receive tubes inserted through them—anathema within the Halsted canon. The patient may also receive external irradiation and chemotherapy to shrink the tumor(s) further.

By this time, you no doubt wonder about the results of a procedure so *truly* radical in the United States. It is the French who have pioneered lumpectomy followed by various radiotherapies, and it is a Frenchman, Dr. Bernard Pierquin of Henri Mondor Hospital in Creteil, outside Paris, who has used the technique on over 500 women since 1961. He has combined it with other radiotherapy and chemotherapy as they developed. He reports a survival rate of 75 percent to 80 percent at ten years—better than much radical mastectomy.

In the United States, Dr. Nisar Syed has done implants since 1973 at Los Angeles County-University of Southern California Medical Center. He reports that a year after treatment, twenty-three of twenty-four patients showed no recurrence of breast cancer. Since a longer test period is obviously needed, Dr. Samuel Hellman, director of the Harvard Joint Center for Radiation Therapy, has followed the progress of at least 150 nonsurgical patients treated with a combination of high-voltage external irradiation and implantation of iridium 192. The patients' conditions ranged from stage I (less than 2 centimeters, no nodal involvement) through stage III (larger than 5 centimeters, with nodal involvement) breast cancers.

According to Dr. Hellman, at two and a half years "there have been no local failures in the stage I and II patients. If there is recurrence, it will take place in 75 percent of patients within two years." Ten patients with nodal involvement at first treatment did develop further tumors.

If you are facing a decision about breast cancer treatment, it should be *your* decision as well as your surgeon's or other physician's. They will proceed to new cases. You—like most women in this book—will live with results of their work. New chemotherapy, new radiotherapy equipment will appear. However, as this chapter shows, very little concerning breast cancer treatment was invented yesterday. If an alternate therapy or surgery interests you, find out about it and do not be intimidated by charges that "it's a fad" or "it hasn't been tried." By this time, everything—plus its combinations—has been tried!

16 / *Irene:*
"I Came Across
as Aggressive"

The setting for my interview with Irene was unusual—the intermission of an open-air dance concert in the twilit greenery of suburban Virginia. We sat high in the theater beside her husband and one of her adult daughters and discussed both her mastectomy and the chemotherapy which she had recently finished.

Irene is a social worker who specializes in programs for counselors working with alcoholics. Fifty-nine years old at the time of the interview, she is the mother of three children—twin girls, age twenty-three, and a son, twenty-six. One of the girls majored in biochemistry and was already working professionally in medical research. Irene's husband, a doctor, is assistant director of one section at the National Cancer Institute, Bethesda, Maryland. As an NCI executive staff member, part of his work involves preparing reports and informing congressional committees on such health issues as environmental pollution and fluoridation of drinking water.

Like the breast history of several women in this book, Irene's first problem was a tumor that proved benign when biopsied. However, her experience of being urged or forced to sign the consent form that allowed simultaneous biopsy and mastectomy, if needed—and not knowing whether she would "wake up with one or two"—had upset her. Thus, in April 1975, when a new problem, a ½-inch inflammation or irritation of one breast, developed, she had determined how much she would allow and the stages at which she would allow it, especially after mammography showed nothing definitive about the irritation.

Women like Irene are making surgeons around the United States rethink their automatic and simultaneous combination of biopsy with mastectomy when a lump proves cancerous. Before the women's movement, doctors may have considered someone like Irene "assertive," "opinionated," "unladylike"—however one describes somebody who's objecting to standard procedure. I would say she is experienced enough to know how much she could cope with, a woman who wanted to make her own body choices and bravely assume responsibility for them.

Doctors state or imply that they do not like whining, dependent patients who want decisions made by others in order to avoid self-responsibility. Yet Irene's doctor did not facilitate her plan to be a more aware kind of patient although at no time did she indicate she would refuse mastectomy if it seemed necessary. If he did investigate the motives behind her decision, the surgeon did not take them seriously enough even to give her a good argument. His objections amounted to "We may not be able to schedule you into the operating room a second time" and "It will be uncomfortable for you to postpone it." Such a ritual assumption that patients can't possibly be trusted to make proper decisions—even when it is they who must live with the results of those decisions—is sad.

Irene felt she would need those ten days between biopsy and mastectomy to adjust psychologically. And she needed the two-stage operation, above all, in order to reduce at any point the uncertainty she had to endure. That she had to bargain also illustrates that doctors' wives don't automatically receive the most cooperative care in town.

The biopsy of the area showing the inflammation was done on an outpatient basis at the Clinical Center, the research hospital on the grounds of National Institutes of Health. (NCI is one of these institutes near Washington, D.C.) When the lab results indicated positive for cancer, mastectomy was scheduled.

Irene's husband confronted his own struggle during

this diagnosis period. Despite (or because of) the fact that he had spent all his professional life, nearly forty years, in medicine and cancer statistics, he found these days a terrifying time. "I felt very threatened," he admitted to me when I completed interviewing him on breast cancer data and trends and he began to relate his wife's experience. He was helped to face the diagnosis by a sympathetic woman colleague who discovered the situation, took the initiative, and invited him to lunch. She said, "I'll bet you didn't know I've had a mastectomy. Here's what your wife will be facing." This compassionate lady also assisted later with practical arrangements and questions about a prosthesis.

I asked, "Did you know, when she phoned, why she was inviting you?"

"No," he replied, "but I went anyway!" He is a handsome, genial man with a sense of humor.

How did other family or friends respond to Irene's situation? She decided to inform some people closest to her at a social event. "At my mother's eightieth birthday party I told the family about the coming biopsy. I told Mother and several friends." Irene telephoned others. "I called my father. I talked with my son. Most people were surprised and just hoped all would go well."

Irene's modified radical mastectomy was performed in June 1975. Unfortunately one underarm lymph node proved positive, which meant she next had to consider and choose among postoperative treatments. "While I was still a patient, about twenty doctors stopped in and invited me to join their different chemotherapy programs." She enrolled in one research project that was testing on postmenopausal women like Irene the effects of various drugs that had proved useful to control cancer in younger women. She was randomly chosen to receive one of three drugs tested in that series.

Many women, including Rose Kushner, author of *Breast Cancer, A Personal History and Investigative Report,* would not and did not tolerate either the delay of multiple paper work or the uncertainty of result that participation in such research entails. Irene, however, sensibly considered her available options: If she refused chemotherapy treatment and had a cancer recurrence, what would she gain? If, with or despite chemotherapy, her cancer also recurred, she'd at least know she'd been brave enough to try what seemed reasonable and possible to help prolong her life. If she had *no* recurrence, then chemotherapy would certainly seem worth suffering, despite its possible side effects. Attempting to predict the future is nearly as maddening as trying to undo the past. She commented, "It was hard because I had no way of knowing, but at least I would be contributing to research *and* feeling I was acting responsibly toward my family and work." The fact that Irene's will was *positively* enlisted in her own care must have influenced in some way the good results that followed.

Her chemotherapy course involved both injections and pills. The doctor probably controlled both dosage and drug carefully because, she noted, "I had very few side effects. I threw up perhaps three times during the eighteen months." When I remarked on her salt-and-pepper hair, cut short and thick, she said, "Well, I saw my scalp for the first time. Some hair fell out after three or four months but it grew back by the end of eighteen months, as you see.

"At the end of each cycle I would feel down, as if I had the flu—just before I received the next injection." Chemotherapy did not interfere with her functioning, in contrast to some cancer patients. "After one injection I drove 350 miles. It just didn't occur to me I couldn't do it." With the end of chemotherapy, Irene's medical regime involved scans of bone and liver every three months for a year, then every six months.

In June 1976, Irene developed a gall bladder problem unrelated to breast or chemotherapy treatment. She was desperate to learn whether this would necessitate her third June in as many years in the hospital; in June 1974 she'd had hip surgery.

Again she met a physician problem. "The doctor was so late for my gall bladder test appointment that I got dressed and left. Later I told him, 'I was ready; you weren't.' " To penalize her, he then refused to give the next test results to her directly. "And I just had to know whether I would be facing another June with a major operation. My attitude was, it's *my* gall bladder—not the doctor's!" She did not have the surgery.

When I asked whether she had sought counseling of any kind to ease her adjustments to surgery and chemotherapy, she described her participation in discussion sessions for cancer patients. "It was a weekly group, unstructured, whose membership constantly changed. It had no goal except it did accomplish a certain sharing of information, and medical personnel were present." Some members merely "griped about doctors' handling of them until I got there and said, 'Look, you can *do* something about your gripes!'

"However, I came across as aggressive. The doctors in the group interpreted my desire to control my own life as a power struggle with them. They didn't like my assuming so much responsibility for my own life!"

Irene's informal and accidental role as group agitator continued. "For instance, while I was in the group, my father died of lung cancer. Naturally I wanted to share this experience because my father died the way he had lived—independent, making his own choices. I told them the truth—that my father hadn't consulted a doctor at all for his lung problem, that he died ten days after one lung collapsed." She agreed he had known of the worsening problem in his throat and lungs but chose, at his advanced age, not to seek treatment. By contrast, Irene sought expert care, both initially and for the follow-up period.

Regardless of how doctors in her counseling group regarded her fighting spirit, which appears aggressive in its own defense when life is at stake, Irene seems exactly the kind of patient Dr. O. Carl Simonton (Chapter 21) would choose to participate in his imagery therapy program. Irene's practical, optimistic spirit ensures that more of her defenses are marshaled into recovering and less into fighting herself. This is positive self-protection in honor of, or search after, active living—rather than negative protection based on fear of death.

About the whole experience she concluded, "After a while you forget the details of mastectomy. The experience fades. My recovery was very rapid from both surgery and chemotherapy. I believe in taking charge of that part of life that's mine."

17 / On Negotiating Mammography, A Doctor, and Consent to Surgery and Treatment

If you feel a high risk for breast cancer, if you must choose a physician for either surgery or more routine breast care, here is what you should know to choose wisely.

Mammography

If mammography is suggested because of your age, particular risk factors, or occurrence of a lump, inquire about the radiation dosage delivered to your breasts by the equipment. Some hospitals and private radiologists have installed new equipment that delivers no more than $1/10$ to $1/4$ rad per exposure, and you should seek this. It is customary to take front and side views of each breast, a total of at least four exposures. You may find more taken if you have small, hard-to-photograph breasts or if error occurs and one or more views do not have adequate resolution. The X ray technician should place a lead apron over your lower ribs and abdomen.

If you receive mammography regularly, ask about availability of thermography or sonography as non-X ray means to visualize your breasts.

Doctor

Gynecologists, although surgeons, ordinarily do not perform breast surgery in this country unless they have completed specialized training. So if you discover a solid lump which your gynecologist or internist decides not to "watch," you will likely see a general surgeon for decisions on the next stage of your care. If he is not an alarmist, if your problem appears benign upon mammography, is likely that a lumpectomy (excisional biopsy) or a needle biopsy (incisional) is all you require.

Discuss whether the lump is positioned in your breast to allow removal under local anesthesia. For this, you are an outpatient, and do not receive general anesthesia nor require a hospital bed. You can go home in a few hours; the laboratory work upon the tumor need not be rushed; and you will save yourself and your insurance company some money.

If, before your biopsy, your doctor(s) are already mentioning possible mastectomy, you will soon learn their mind-set upon the topic.

If you are agreeable to mastectomy (probably modified radical), should cancer be found, ask about:

• A two-stage operation (lumpectomy separated from mastectomy). This avoids the hasty frozen-section biopsy performed while you are anesthetized and allows you a few days to adjust psychologically to what is occurring.
• Preoperative and postoperative drugs, side effects of surgery, and whether Reach to Recovery works in your area.
• What further treatment or tests your doctor plans or does, such as chest X rays, bone scans. The new test for whether a cancer is estrogen-dependent, for example, requires fresh tissue within a few hours of surgery.
• His opinions on radiotherapy, kinds of chemotherapy, and who administers these in your area.
• Having a family member included in future explanations and decisions.

If your surgeon admits he performs few breast operations (four to five mastectomies per year) or if his answers to reasonable questions amount to, "I'm taking it out. What more do you need to know?" seek another surgeon. Say that you desire a further opinion.

When a mastectomy is performed skillfully by an experienced surgeon, there is little or no permanent postoperative swelling. The underarm lymph nodes are removed in bloc (in continuous section) for analysis during both radical and modified radical mastectomy. Following this, the lymph ducts or vessels, which are also cut in or around the node area, must be rejoined carefully to allow an uninterrupted flow of lymphatic fluid from the hand through the arm toward the heart. If they are poorly realigned, severe or prolonged arm and shoulder swelling results. This is one reason that women who agree to a mastectomy should seek a surgeon with much experience or specialization in breast work. By one 1966 estimate (J. H. Farrow, "Rehabilitation Following Radical Breast Surgery," *Cancer* 16:222), 25 percent of patients develop "moderate lymphedema" (swelling) and 10 percent "marked lymphedema." Obviously many mastectomies are still not done as skillfully as possible.

Competent follow-up care to mastectomy is crucial to your psychological and physical recovery. If the tone of your early doctor-patient negotiations is poor, this does not bode well for speedy recovery, let alone guiding you through the traumas of waiting and surgery.

If you are too upset to pursue *any* of these matters during your initial visit, arrange another appointment or at least a phone call to gain further information. If you are a premenopausal woman, your doctor will probably want to reexamine your breasts after your next menstrual period, giving you further time to regroup your forces.

If you desire an alternative to radical mastectomy, such as lumpectomy or partial mastectomy, do not postpone seeking treatment. It *is* possible to discover competent surgeons who will do lesser procedures, but you, like Veronica Gardos (Chapter 18), must persevere in discovering them.

If diet therapy or a psychological approach to cancer to help strengthen your body or cope with stress interests you, it is best to combine this with at least a lumpectomy so that you know definitely whether you have breast cancer and what kind of breast cancer you do have. After a lumpectomy your body has that much less disease to cope with.

Remember this paradox about cancer: While there

are no "miracle cures," there are millions who are cured—alive and well. Compared to lung or pancreatic cancer, for example, breast cancer is both treatable and curable—provided you seek competent care early.

Treatment Consent Forms

One reason for discussing procedures carefully with your doctor is that you need time to evaluate the wording that will later appear on the consent form. If this important document is presented by a secretary or a nurse for your hurried signature a few hours before surgery, it is probably too late at that point to negotiate or even to question.

It is your doctor's responsibility to word surgical procedures in language understandable to you. If you do not understand it, you are not giving what is called in legal terminology "informed consent."

The first clause of such a form usually gives your surgeon and his assistants the right to perform "necessary services to include the following procedures." Here he will probably handwrite in what you and he have discussed, "lumpectomy, biopsy, possible modified radical mastectomy"—if you have agreed to this third subject. If you have not, it should not appear on the form.

Never sign a blank form.

Specifying the procedures that are less than a radical mastectomy helps limit and demystify the later clauses in the average consent form. Examples are: the right of your doctor and other hospital personnel to administer anesthesia, intravenous medications, other drugs, blood transfusions; the right to extend original procedures into remedying "all conditions that require treatment and are not known to the above physicians at the time the procedure(s) is commenced."

At some point, the average form also states that the nature, purpose, risks, complications, and possible alternate treatments have been explained to you and that you "fully understand the consent given herein." In desperation before a biopsy, I once wrote on a consent form: "Nature of the disease is too uncertain at this point for this clause to be true."

The final clause will probably remind you that "the

practice of medicine and surgery is not an exact science" and that "no guarantee or assurance has been made or implied as to the beneficial results that may be obtained as a result of the procedure(s)."

Confrontation with such enlarged self-protection for your doctor plus the hospital and its personnel should make you realize why your consent is no mere clerical detail. I believe a revised form is needed to state that under certain conditions (for example, presence of a benign tumor), you agree only to a lumpectomy and biopsy of the tissue obtained. If cancer is discovered, you should be given a later chance to negotiate a renewed consent based on fresh knowledge—size, kind, position of your tumor(s), results of further tests. If evidence indicates that cancer has already spread beyond the breast, doctors in some medical centers perform only a lumpectomy, then proceed immediately to radiotherapy or chemotherapy. Such doctors would not require your immediate consent to mastectomy.

To avoid consulting a lawyer before or afterward, you can solve many problems by asking nurses, patients, hospital volunteers to locate a doctor who is negotiable in the first place. The gynecologist who recommends you, for example, to a general surgeon knows quite well how his colleague will handle your case, depending on the extent and nature of your disease. Pry this information from the gynecologist before consulting the new doctor.

Remember: *Any decisions you do not make or participate in will be made for you*—unless you demonstrate the ability to cope, reason, and choose among possibilities.

18 / *Veronica Gardos: Achieving a Choice*

Veronica Gardos is a young woman who believed "I was a candidate for less than a total mastectomy." Born in Australia, she lives in Manhattan although her work takes her often to California and across the Pacific to China. She is a consultant to U.S. cosmetic and fashion companies for the export of fashion accessories to the Far East.

Negotiating with various Australian surgeons for lumpectomy and partial mastectomy, she "got a few responses that amounted to 'Why don't you return to America with your women's lib ideas?' "

In April 1977 she was en route to Australia and Hong Kong via Los Angeles when she accidentally discovered a lump in the upper outer quadrant of her right breast. "When I came up from the swimming pool, I walked past the mirror in my friend's house. I thought I saw a piece of dirt or soot on my breast. I tried to wipe it off. It didn't wipe off." She was thirty-six years old.

She consulted a California surgeon with a large breast practice. Since the lump was small (1.2 centimeters) and appeared benign upon mammography, the surgeon tried aspirating it. Veronica had a history of benign disease. "I had lumpy breasts." In the few years from her twenty-ninth to thirty-sixth birthdays she had mammography ten times; all problems had proved benign.

157

This time the lump would not aspirate.

She phoned her family doctor in Australia—later described as "my one mistake"—to alert him that she was arriving in Sydney with what everybody assumed would be another benign problem.

She negotiated with him for a biopsy (lumpectomy). The first shock came when the tumor proved malignant. Since she wanted the opinion of more than one pathologist, she requested results of the paraffin section examination of the tumor, completed a few days after the frozen section. It, too, indicated malignancy.

The next shock came when she began negotiating further treatment and met outrage and suspicion at the idea of a woman with breast cancer receiving anything less than radical mastectomy. Even the nurses said, "Do what the doctors tell you. They'll do right by you. They know more than you do."

One of the hospital surgeons visited her room with the family doctor who had performed the biopsy. She wanted to learn their recommendation but got annoyed when the family doctor announced he was leaving the room to discuss her case with the other physician. She asked, "Why are you leaving when I'm paying you to discuss my case with me?" She added to me, "He didn't start out being negative. He was nice, but still went outside." It soon became apparent he, too, favored radical mastectomy.

"While in the hospital, I asked various breast surgeons to come to my room and explain possible treatment," she continued. "I thought I was a candidate for less than a total mastectomy." One of these men, a cancer surgeon with a special interest in breast treatment, is professor of cancer education at an institute at the University of Sydney. Veronica described him as "the head of professional breast surgery in Australia." He proved interested in her case—and negotiable regarding treatment. "He thought I'd be a candidate for a partial, with lymph glands also removed. I gave him permission to do a total mastectomy, but he knew I preferred a partial. We had a gentlemen's agreement." She agreed to lymph gland removal. "I wanted to know that it hadn't spread there. If it had, certainly a more radical operation was indicated."

A man in his mid-sixties with decades of surgical experience, the surgeon negotiated politely with her. He even investigated survival results of partial mastectomy in medical literature (research from Italy and Guy's Hospital, London). She described him as "a special man" and termed the process "a decision we arrived at together."

Only *one percent* of mastectomy for cancer in Australia, as in this country, is partial.

During her second surgery a few days later, he removed an upper outer segment of the right breast beneath the skin plus all the right underarm nodes. None of the nodes proved cancerous. "I believe time will prove in selected cases that partial mastectomy is a correct and effective surgery," Veronica said.

She described her hospital care as "excellent. I had lovely nurses, but none of them had ever seen a partial mastectomy. The rumor got around the hospital that I had refused all mastectomy. When it came time for the unveiling, I was very nervous. It was scheduled for 12 noon, then for 2 P.M. I knew a woman at ten years afterward who can't look at her breast. I wanted to know and yet I had trouble looking." One of the day nurses, who also had never seen this combination of partial mastectomy with node removal for cancer, took the bandages off bit by bit, "gently, lovingly. Now this piece, now that piece," Veronica recalled.

When I inquired about family's or friends' attitudes, she answered, "They helped by behaving well. No one cried or carried on. They were confused by my wanting something different from the normal. My sisters and friends supported me. They knew it was important to me. Everybody was happy for me that they'd found my cancer, that I'd had the operation I'd wanted. Nobody who comes in and weeps does the patient a service.

"The patient herself has to create the environment. The leadership came from me. I had troubles, but I was going to overcome them. I never cried or got hysterical. I knew I couldn't get hysterical because I was commander. If I showed weakness, they were going to get me. I was fighting for life and breast."

While still in Australia, she found notice of her medical iconoclasm spreading. Radio and television shows asked her to appear and state her reasons for the lesser surgery. She wrote some articles, and she and the breast surgeon made a videotape for medical education on the need for two-stage operations and for counseling patients during all phases and decisions.

In a tape made for Australian radio her surgeon said, "Veronica was a young woman with a mobile lump [usually indicates benign tumor]. There is no need for a woman in this situation to go to sleep without knowing whether she will lose a breast." Since eight of ten lumps prove benign, Veronica added that the two-stage operation "relieves 80 percent of women of the need *ever* to face mastectomy—and it gives the woman with breast cancer a few days to choose the doctor she wants. Otherwise, a woman wakes up thinking they got the lump when actually she had the breast removed."

Her recovery period was complicated by the fact that business travel through Australia and to Hong Kong did not allow her an opportunity to pursue the correct physiotherapy, and what she received she described as "incorrect." The hospital physiotherapist visited her room and gave her exercises "too strenuous for my condition. 'The more you do, the better you'll get.' " Veronica, believing her, exercised enthusiastically. Out of the hospital her shoulder remained swollen. At first she thought the discomfort psychosomatic, but finally "it was painful to write. I blamed lack of communication." The doctor hadn't directly informed the physiotherapist what he had done. Lacking the complete technical vocabulary, Veronica explained insufficiently to the physiotherapist and left Australia with inappropriate exercises.

She returned to work half-days at first. "I really missed only two days of my life, two days when I didn't feel too great." She thought by four weeks after surgery she'd be on her way through Australia again to Hong Kong.

Finally her shoulder froze from pain and phlebitis. "I thought it was cancer of the shoulder." With daily massage and correct exercise by a physiotherapist back in Manhattan, however, she regained full motion. Her fear lessened.

She showed me her breast scar—a horizontal white line against the tan on her upper right breast—and photos of herself again in a two-piece bathing suit with her family in

Australia. Her right underarm, even beneath a jersey top, looked normal also. In addition, the physiotherapist suggested "I go home and play tennis. I did and it was the greatest thing in the world."

She has continued to inform both her Australian surgeon and the Los Angeles doctor of her progress. She described the Los Angeles surgeon in two words: "He cared."

I asked further how she had coped with negative emotions surrounding her total experience. First we discussed fear. "I haven't coped with it yet," she said. "It's still in my life. . . . I didn't have a radical mastectomy so I didn't have the traditional anger. I felt anger that I had to fight to achieve civilized care. I vented it. A two-stage operation should at least be suggested to all women in this predicament.

"I'm an activist. I didn't feel helpless. I had to be in control, partaker of my fate. I had an intense desire to get things done properly." She joked, "When I get my hair cut, I can choose the length. I consider my breast at least as important as my hair!

"I developed over the years into a person who handles her own affairs. Cancer is just another aspect of life. It's a matter of personality how one copes with the challenges it presents." She described a recent incident involving a winter plane flight that detoured her and 300 other passengers from New York, where they wanted to land, to the Washington, D.C. airport. Some passengers were confused or helpless at the changed plans. Veronica, used to travel contingencies, went about booking herself and others into hotel rooms upon landing.

When I asked whether she remembered anything particularly comforting that speeded her recovery, she told me an incident involving a courageous California designer of jersey fashions for women. Veronica had heard that at a recent style show this designer, Harriet Selwyn, had personally descended the show's runway in a snug-fitting item. To the gaze of customers, reporters, and other designers, the garment revealed that Harriet Selwyn now had—only one breast.

Veronica added, "I had never worn a bra. After the partial mastectomy, however, I started wearing one and stuffed it with whatever." When she heard about Harriet

Selwyn's example, she stopped wearing the bra. Self-consciousness decreased. "She, without knowing it, did a terrific thing for me. We have to get women who've had breast cancer out of the closet," she emphasized.

On a radio tape which I heard, Veronica and her Australian surgeon discussed aspects of breast cancer care with Rose Kushner and another mastectomee. When the conversation verged into how to resume sexual life and tell a lover the facts of breast cancer or surgery, Veronica's doctor said that Australian women "very seldom" asked him about sexual relations following mastectomy. Veronica set a common urban scene involving an unmarried couple who share cocktails, dinner, coffee, liqueur, and . . . bed. Given this dating situation, when should a woman tell the man of her breast cancer or mastectomy? "There should be some time between the liqueur and bed," the doctor admitted. "Or between the coffee and liqueur," Veronica decided. "Partial mastectomy has not affected my sex life. It has made no difference at all."

Rose Kushner believes that telling another human being about one's experience strengthens a woman and helps her cope. She has estimated that only about one-half of approximately 700,000 U.S. mastectomees (NCI Biometry Branch statistic) want even friends to know. "The other women are unreachable. Jacqueline Susann died fourteen years postmastectomy, and not even her friends knew. We have to reach women who sit in the house and feel less than human, let alone less than women."

When I interviewed Veronica, she had resumed her full life of meetings, phone calls, writing merchandise orders, travel. In the United States, as in Australia, when she reveals her surgery at doctors' offices, the response is apt to be, "Where did you get *that*? How did you manage *that* one?" as if by negotiating a conservative surgery, she is some kind of radical. Another paradox of breast cancer. . . .

She merely repeats, "My doctor and I discussed, and both came to agreement about a lifesaving, tailor-made operation."

COPING

19 / Coping with Breast Cancer and Mastectomy

You never stop worrying.   —RITA, five years after surgery

The only way I do as well as I do is to deny the whole thing.
                              —NATALIA, five years after surgery

I remember crying with anger and frustration.
                              —ELISE, three years after surgery

A truism about cancer states that the treatment is worse than the disease. Certainly while radical mastectomy remains the treatment of necessity, not of choice, for breast cancer, as much of a woman's initial cope-ability is needed to confront mutilation as to live with the dilemma of cancer itself. Assuming skillful surgery, an individual's personality, rather than age, determines her ability to recover from the physical and psychological effects of mastectomy.

Both doctors and patients are likely to assume that a woman past menopause will not miss a breast. Joan Fromewick, a medical social worker at Montefiore Hospital, Bronx, New York, told me of an incident from one of her counseling groups. A woman in her sixties, trying to cheer a younger patient, remarked, "I'm old. My breast doesn't matter. But you, you're a young woman with all your life ahead of you."

A woman in her seventies interrupted, "Speak for

yourself! I'm seventy-two, and I feel I've lost a good friend."

Ms. Fromewick commented, "That woman was great. We liked her so much. She had so much *spirit.*"

Researchers agree that a woman copes or fails to cope with mastectomy based on how much it deranges or destroys her basic character defenses. These are habitual patterns of behavior that satisfy needs, maintain safety and security, meet demands of the environment. Research psychiatrist Dr. Morton Bard summarized, "The impact of breast amputation will depend less on a woman's age than upon the character adaptations disrupted by it." Two psychiatrists I questioned believed a woman responds to breast cancer or surgery as she has to other life crises or stresses. Veronica Gardos' level-headed statements (Chapter 18), for instance, support this idea.

Before the mastectomy, a woman feels a natural anxiety related to surgery and anesthesia plus the specifically feminine reaction to a future minus a breast. Fear of anesthesia seems to relate to the horror of being reduced to childhood helplessness or vulnerability. Certainly general anesthesia tests one's trust. As one patient put it: "Even if you're in good hands, you have no control whatever. You're out and can't do anything at all."

Fueled by sedatives and anesthesia, dreams during the crisis or surgery can be terrifying. They, too, recall childhood nightmares. A waking preoccupation with breasts translates into sleep images like these.

I just dream about my breasts. I dreamt that I saw a row of what I thought were breasts. They were all distorted. I thought I was in a butcher shop and they were hung up on hooks like meat all around me.

I was walking down the gangplank of a ferryboat with a lot of other women. At the bottom of the gangplank was a man and he was checking each woman to see if she had her breasts. I was getting closer to the bottom when I woke up.

Ferrymen, of course, are ancient, mythic figures who conduct humans to another world. Are surgeons and anesthesiologists their contemporary counterpart?

I was taking this little girl to a store and bought her a new pair of shoes. After leaving the store we were waiting for a trolley car on a street near an open field. There was a cow in the field, and as we waited, I noticed that the little girl's shoes were deep in mud. As I bent down to clean the shoes, the cow came toward us and when I looked up it was eating a hole in the top of the child's head. I woke up screaming and I've been very upset since then. It was horrible. I can't forget it. I wasn't able to relax in the hospital after that.

Does it surprise you that such dreams are considered normal? They also appear during pregnancy, another period of rapid body alteration culminating in hospitalization.

Defense mechanisms, activated or reactivated by surgery, prove inadequate for some women. They later regret and resent their involuntary consent to mastectomy. Months afterward, one wrote:

Why did I ever go and have this done? . . . My sister and all the relatives tell me to forget. It's easy to say. They told me they were going to take it out, but they took the whole thing off. I never would have let them. I'm even ashamed to walk down the street. . . . Everything is changed; I even have blotches all over my face now. You're going to say, "You're married, so why are you worried?" It's not that. I'm still conscious of it.

In this matter of mourning a lost body image, feeling "half man, half woman," Shirley Temple Black wrote:

I don't want to leave the impression that the whole thing is at all easy. It is an ugly operation, a maiming operation, and there is a certain amount of physical pain. I'm not yet comfortable in my revised body. My left arm hurts from the shoulder to the elbow. I seem to be off balance, and as I look in the mirror I feel quite unattractive. . . . I will accommodate to the look and to the feel. My arm hurts less each day, and my mirror looks back at me more kindly.

Like other public personalities, Shirley Temple Black received many letters—approximately 50,000—following her mastectomy. The writers' concern helped, but her words speak what any woman feels.

Many women report a sense of life standing still or

surrealistically dividing into "before" and "after" the facts of cancer and treatment. Some find concentration or future planning impossible, until immediate crises abate and they dare to hope again.

A few women may see loss of a breast as a magnification of "what's awful in life" (Judy's phrase—Chapter 20) or as punishment for sexual activity engaged in many years ago. According to Drs. Morton Bard and Arthur Sutherland of the Research Psychiatry Section at Sloan-Kettering, one patient who should be watched and helped is the woman whose demeanor amounts to manic-depression.

. . . patients may appear elated, unconvincingly cheerful, talkative, and physically overactive. Elation, usually characterized by these manifestations, is a fragile mask for a serious depression. One such patient became profoundly depressed at the time of diagnosis. A week later she exhibited marked overactivity and brittle cheerfulness. She flippantly expressed the belief that she would die in surgery. During her postoperative course she manifested a hypochondriacal depression.

Betty Rollin, author of *First, You Cry,* apparently experienced a period like this. In a radio interview she described herself before mastectomy: "I thought I wanted to know exactly whether the doctor planned mastectomy, but I didn't. The doctor said, '50 percent chance.' If he'd said, '99 percent,' I couldn't have taken it anyway. The doctor wisely evaluated me." She described herself in the hospital as "artificially jolly, terrific, joking," followed by, "You come home and suddenly it hits you."

Male Response to Mastectomy

It seems unfair to have to worry about that, too.

—MASTECTOMY PATIENT

I think the hottest place in hell should be reserved for men who might make a wife feel she is any less of a woman, because it's not true at all.

—MARVELLA BAYH

Husbands leave you in droves, and friends leave in droves. Not just from loss of a breast but from fear that cancer is contagious.
—WOMAN RECOVERED FROM BREAST CANCER

Do husbands or menfriends leave in droves?

As far as I know, no survey on this topic exists (perhaps just as well), so answers vary here according to whether the respondents are optimistic or not about their love relationships and their recovery from surgery.

Dr. Eugene Thiessen of New York University Medical Center and the Strang Clinic, Manhattan, gave an answer that encompassed several possibilities and presented what a concerned surgeon can do to ease a tense situation. "All women are apprehensive about self-image and how mastectomy will affect their attractiveness to a new mate, the other sex. Some husbands I know have disappeared, never to be seen again. Breast cancer is a family disease. I encourage the whole family to come in. One couple said, 'After seven years a woman needs reassurance, but mastectomy hasn't lessened our relationship.' "

Sometimes the very woman most shattered, least able to cope, with mastectomy may be least likely to get help because involvement in her care seems too threatening in the face of such total need. Husbands, lovers, friends *do* fail temporarily or permanently while they endure their own struggles. "He told me my scar was downright ugly." "My husband is an alcoholic, and this was just one more thing he couldn't handle." "Only people who are full of hate get tumors." These comments are intended to air other grudges in already fragile relationships.

The challenge is to continue to love someone who seems rejecting—or at least not to reject *him* in turn because one's own self-esteem has plummeted. One women expressed it: "I was reluctant to marry after the mastectomy although I was going with a man at the time." A wife said, "My fear of rejection was so great that I turned it around and rejected Dan." A fifty-one-year-old California woman said, "It was the worst thing that could possibly happen. I felt shattered for my husband, ashamed, degraded."

Dr. Marc Schwartz, a Connecticut psychiatrist who

counsels on mastectomy-related problems, estimated that only 5 to 10 percent of couples have major marital problems following surgery. Another 20 percent have moderate difficulties in readjustment. In 1977, Dr. Schwartz reported three questions afflicting most husbands: (1) Will she live? (2) How can I help her? (3) What about sex? (third on the list). "Even six months later," noted Dr. Schwartz, "men seem much less concerned than women with the physical and sexual aspects of the operation."

If these men were responding honestly, this may be another area where some men and women live at cross purposes, failing to communicate. Dr. Schwartz termed such false assumptions "a misreading that is interpreted as rejection."

Dr. Mildred Hope Witkin is a psychotherapist with the Human Sexuality Program at Payne Whitney Clinic, Manhattan. The survivor of breast cancer and two mastectomies, one in the 1950s, the other in 1974, she told a story of how she and her husband, instead of following their feelings, followed some inappropriate advice. During her first hospitalization a psychiatrist of the least-said-soonest-mended philosophy advised Dr. Witkin's husband to act as if nothing had happened, to display "no concern or special caring." When the young husband did this, his wife concluded he no longer loved her. She admitted it took many years to repair the damage. For the second operation, however, "This time we were able to find unexpected strengths in ourselves and in our relationship."

The amount of help a woman gets from her husband or friends depends on the prior quality of the relationships. And *it is often she who must set the tone for how to cope*, what to do. As several women in this book emphasize, she must provide would-be helpers with intelligible clues to what she needs or wants. A general rule, which surgeons are admitting only slowly, is that *husbands, lovers, children who feel included* in medical explanations of diagnosis and treatment *receive*, first, some help with their own fears or ignorance and, second, *the best chance to prove useful and capable*. Shrouding cancer in secrecy, evading family members, recognizing but two extremes—ignoring a woman's emotions or overprotecting her—any of these stances impedes communication and help. Some post-mastectomy counseling groups (see Chapter 21) now encourage male participation.

The following comment from a New York teacher following her mastectomy summarizes the average male's ambivalence. "My husband's mother died of cancer. At times my husband was supportive to me. At other times I felt like killing him. He walked around patting me on the shoulder and looked like he would cry. After I came from surgery, he was surprised I was still alive. . . . What helped me was that he had no qualms about looking at me, at the scar."

Many husbands and lovers, after initial shock, respond nobly. Shirley Temple Black wrote of her husband, "His love is without sham, a love that does not look aside. It is direct, constant, and strong." Another California woman wrote after mastectomy, "I was alive! As for my husband, he took me on a second honeymoon." One social worker reported, "Breast cancer is a terrible disease, but I've been amazed at how resilient people are. They really *do* cope. Their lives are *not* devastated. We just don't see broken marriages and other terrible problems. The men are usually very supportive." One wife described a marriage anyone would envy because it summarizes the whole miracle of healing.

It sounds funny but he's always been like a girl friend to me. Every evening that summer we sat in the living room, had a glass of wine, and talked. We discussed all my fears and he made me realize I hadn't been singled out. Sexually, he's always been a warm person. He built me up. He made me feel I would get well and we'd be together . . . and sex just followed. What can I tell you? He restored my soul.

Although a woman's support system need not, and usually does not, depend on whether she is married, the single, divorced, or widowed woman coping with loneliness or aging seems more devastated by breast cancer and mastectomy. Yet any woman who turns to her surgeon for help with confronting and controlling her own feelings may not find it. If she does not, here are a few reasons why.

A Surgeon's Emotions

According to Dr. Reuven Snyderman, a New Jersey plastic surgeon who performs breast reconstructions (Chapter 23), "Surgeons feel guilt when they discover cancer." However, in one psychiatrist's words, they also tend to be "professionally immunized to the impact of surgery on others."

Some surgeons, like some husbands, naturally and sympathetically offer what patients need during crises. Judy (Chapter 20) enjoyed such a surgeon. "He makes time for questions, is explicit, doesn't talk above a layperson's head. He's always available, a dedicated physician. He's a specialist but also a whole person."

Many patients, who never experience such skill or compassion, thirst for it as for a cure to the disease itself. Georgia Photopoulos is a woman asked by the Chicago ACS to develop a pilot program to meet the nonphysical needs of patients and families. It is called CANCER CALL-PAC; the final abbreviation stands for "People Against Cancer." Here is part of her story:

I was 34 years old when I discovered I had cancer. . . . I have had to draw on every ounce of my energy at my command to wage this six-year battle. During this time I have undergone bilateral mastectomy with metastasis to the lymph nodes, a recurrence, 120 treatments of cobalt . . . many localized excisions in the throat, right axilla, ribs, oophorectomy, and a medical hysterectomy. . . .

I discovered that fear is the greatest enemy. Fearing cancer is harder than having it. Fear is what makes you delay in seeking treatment, fear is what cripples your ability to deal with it, and fear ultimately can be fatal.

I think that doctors and nurses could do a lot to help cancer patients accept and deal with their diagnosis by explaining things a little better. They should explain what procedures will be followed, that pain is normal following surgery. . . . I think that some doctors withhold information from patients on the assumption that they might not be able to take it, or they assume that someone else will explain the hard facts of the case to the patient. Following my first mastectomy, whenever I had questions concerning the surgery, the gynecologist referred me to the surgeon, who in turn referred me back to the gynecologist, and then on to the radiologist. It was only by accident that I stumbled onto the information that there had been metastasis in the underarm lymph nodes.

It is the patient's right to know where the trouble is, what it is, and what has to be done to provide a cure. . . .

I feel I represent the countless thousands of cancer patients, the unheard voices pleading for an empathetic ear, a measure of understanding, and a sense of direction.

In 1978, after five years' treatment that a Californian, Louise Crossley, considered worse than the disease, she called out her friends and relatives to picket her doctor's office to obtain records and cease her medical care. Of her doctor's decision that she remain uninformed about her own case, she observed, "If they hand you a deck of forty-eight cards and tell you to play solitaire, you can't win!" During a radio interview Rose Kushner remarked, "It's easier to get information from the CIA than from the medical profession."

Like other occupations, medicine draws to it people of particular character types, which psychiatrists (M.D.s themselves) have researched. Dr. Andrew Watson of the University of Michigan said in a *New York Times* interview, "They are selected for their test-taking ability and they frequently are incapable of coping with the basic requirement of their professions: counseling clients or patients. Many of them hate such counseling. And they feel guilty that they do."

Someone else quipped, "Medical students begin with a corpse and work up. What does that tell you about their value system?"

Dr. Richard Selzer, a general surgeon on the Yale School of Medicine faculty, defends himself this way in *Mortal Lessons, Notes on the Art of Surgery:*

It is the nature of creatures to live within a cuirass that is both their constriction and their protection. The carapace of the turtle is his fortress and retreat, yet keeps him writhing on his back in the sand. So is the surgeon rendered impotent by his own empathy and compassion. The surgeon cannot weep. When he cuts the flesh, his own must not bleed. Here it is all work. Like an asthmatic hungering for air, longing to take just one deep breath, the surgeon struggles not to feel. It is suffocating to press the feeling out. It would be easier to weep or mourn. . . .

Breast cancer patients, including some I interviewed, too often conclude it is their fault if doctors do not show more interest even in legitimate topics like postsurgical recovery or diet to maintain energy. Others expect surgeons to work magic against emotions they themselves cannot confront or handle. However, as normally functioning adults, many merely want *help*—cues—for how to cope in a sensible way.

And if it involves tears. . . . One postmastectomy patient I heard joked about Betty Rollin's title, "It should be *First, You Cry . . . Second, You Cry . . . Third, You Cry."* No need for elaborate theories about mourning body image. The point is that both women used the tears to begin surviving and functioning again.

Now that the women's movement and many consumer health groups have exposed "paternalized" medicine, a few physicians have publicly confessed their errors—and emerged humbler, wiser for the experience. Dr. Arthur Holleb, a former breast surgeon, now an ACS vice-president, wrote:

I thought I had been doing a pretty good job of providing the pat on the back, the reassuring, "Don't worry, dear, everything will be like it was before." Little did I know! Most of us who specialized in breast surgery apparently did not recognize that much more assistance could be given to women who had lost a breast.

20 / Judy: "It's Easier for Younger Patients"

Judy and her welcoming committee—seven eager, curious house pets—met me in the living room of her Manhattan apartment. It was one of those welcomes when it's hard to know where to focus—on Judy in her plum-colored jump suit, on the white toy poodles, on the pride of cats, large and small. Judy had salvaged some of them from extinction on New York streets. Gradually she herded them all under control. They distributed themselves on the two sofas to scrutinize our interview—and attack the milk for our coffee.

Judy's husband, a percussionist who was on concert tour, called during the interview because Judy had been hospitalized the week before with an asthma attack. Judy's daughter, Betsy, described as "nine years old, going on seventy-three. She's like a grandmother," wandered in from school while we talked.

Forty-three at the time of our interview, Judy found a lump during a breast self-examination she had done four years previously. Indeed, she seemed one of the few women I interviewed whose tumor discovery was not accidental, who practiced such self-monitoring regularly *before* a problem developed. It was a small lump in the upper outer quadrant, the most common site where 41 percent of reported breast cancer occurs. (Another 34 percent attacks the nipple area.) In the left breast, this quadrant is called the "one to three o'clock" position.

When she saw her gynecologist, he suggested waiting—but only until after her next period. Soft and movable like a benign growth, the lump persisted. Her gynecologist next suggested a breast surgeon. "Both of them thought it was nothing," Judy recalled. She signed only the biopsy form without coercion toward anything further.

The biopsied lump proved to be cancer of a rare, noninvasive, nonmetastasizing kind. Unfortunately, only 2 percent to 10 percent of breast cancers are such *comedo carcinoma*. Its internal substance resembles the sebum found in blackheads. It is also a form of carcinoma *in situ*, since the cancer cells have unbroken membranes and the tumor is encapsulated by normal tissue.

However, because it was cancer, Judy had to consider further therapy. Her father, a surgeon with contacts at a teaching hospital, gathered information for her, but neither he nor the surgeon pressured her. "They gave me the option of further treatment. I could have had radiation instead of mastectomy. I didn't want to take the gamble. I wanted the best chance possible for survival."

Judy's surgery was a modified radical mastectomy of the left breast. Her breast surgeon "is everybody's dream of what a doctor and surgeon should be. He makes time for questions, is explicit, doesn't talk above a layperson's head. He's always available, a dedicated physician. He's a specialist but also a *whole person*," she emphasized.

Judy experienced "no unusual physical problems." Her psychological difficulties also seemed moderate; she is a warm, emotional person used to expressing feelings. She first described herself as "appalled" that breast surgery should be so "routine."

I asked about her family's and friends' attitudes. "I told Betsy right away, three or four days postoperative. She helped by attaching and detaching my Hemovac apparatus so we could walk around. She's still involved. I do test-wearing of different prostheses and products. She tells me what looks good or bad. Now she calls me 'the star of breast cancer.'" Since recovery, Judy has appeared on television and radio with Mary (Chapter 22) and Dr. Philip Strax, a specialist in mammography and early detection.

"How children react is determined by how parents react. Children project their mother's attitude toward breast cancer. My family and friends were sympathetic and supportive. Because of my friends, both men and women, I had no negative memories."

Judy remained hospitalized ten days because her home life was strenuous. Besides five-year-old Betsy, she and her husband were foster-parenting two teenage boys.

"I immediately returned to work. Mastectomy caused me no problems in marriage that weren't preexisting."

Judy did confess her "only negative feeling that was disruptive," her "one moment of superpanic," that arrived during an airplane trip six months postsurgery. "I guess I had six months' residue of fear of not being cured, fear of recurrence, that needed discharging." After driving long hours through California mountains, Judy had a case of tense neck muscles before her flight. Seeking interesting reading, she bought a paperback copy of Robert Anderson's novel *After*. The story of a man whose wife dies of breast cancer (Judy discovered too late), it opens with a scene in which the woman is bedridden with neck pain from metastasized cancer. Judy's reading choice, plus her stiff neck, rooted her in her seat. "I taste that panic still," she recalled. "I felt like tearing my skin off."

Desperate for diversion, she tried to socialize with the man next to her, only to discover he was a psychiatrist with a morbid fear of flying. He was planning, he announced, to gulp two martinis and fall asleep as fast as possible.

On her own resources Judy made it through the flight. Her aching neck, which proved no more serious than muscle spasm, soon ended.

She continued, "My greatest problem was finding a prosthesis that was comfortable," that would look good under the leotards she wears for music rehearsals. A helpful employee of Regenesis, one of New York's postmastectomy shops (Chapter 23), sewed a special prosthesis for Judy—a customized pocket bra that held the silicone form. "I looked and felt comfortable again." Judy's breasts are small, and she regularly wears backless, strapless garments that other women might need only in summer.

When Mary, coordinator of Manhattan Reach to Recovery volunteers, recommended Judy as a prosthesis model, Judy continued her search for new equipment. She showed me several she had test-worn, including Second Nature, which has an interesting history.

In 1970 a mastectomee happened to describe her problems with uncomfortable, unattractive prostheses to a Philadelphia sculptor. She wanted something ready-made for the right or left side that didn't look "like a beanbag or a triangle."

The sculptor fashioned appropriate models in plaster and clay and showed them to a class. Two of his students, entrepreneurs in the bicycle rack business, saw a good idea, made further molds and designs, and contracted with two more partners, including a European chemist who formulated both the soft outer skin and the special glue used with Second Nature.

Judy commented, "Many prostheses of the silicone gel variety are guaranteed only two to three years because the gel softens. Every day, oil in it migrates outward onto a woman's skin. Second Nature has a skin that is both nonpermeable and doesn't irritate with rough edges. It has a darker, nippled area and with the glue, I've worn it braless under a silk shirt. I can wear it with confidence even under a maillot [tank suit]. I've slept, dived, showered, and worn it for many days at a time glued on. And if I want to wear a strapless, backless dress, it's lighter than other models so I don't have to look for a built-in bra that can hold the weight of other prostheses." Second Nature can also be worn unglued by inserting it into the pocket of the usual postmastectomy bra.

Fully half my interview with Judy involved her views on integrating the mastectomy and cancer experiences into one's life and on her work as a Reach to Recovery volunteer. She now visits seven to ten patients a week because "I felt the need for younger women in Reach to Recovery and because I'm willing to travel all over Manhattan, including up to Harlem Hospital, not just to hospitals near this apartment."

Judy is thoroughly optimistic about the younger

woman's recovery. "It's easier for younger patients. Provided, of course, that a woman does not have systemic disease, she can recover easily if she does not let the breast become a scapegoat for preexisting problems, for what's awful in life. With today's rules what they are, I also get along well with single women."

She told another anecdote on herself. "At the time of mastectomy I was warned about possible depression. So I dutifully made appointments with a psychiatrist." When the depression didn't materialize, after several months he suggested she come back only if she needed to. "Well, it's four years later, and I'm still waiting for the depression!" In contrast to older women, retired or widowed, Judy's energetic life-style that includes a husband and young daughter is certainly one reason for her buoyancy.

I inquired who, in Judy's opinion and based on her Reach to Recovery counseling, experiences more difficult physical or psychological recovery from the trauma of surgery and "living with the diagnosis," as Rita calls it. Judy mentioned first "the older group, or anyone who has been conditioned to the idea that cancer is synonymous with death." In the 1930s, for example, fewer than 20 percent of all cancer patients survived even five years.

The second part of her answer was nearly identical with one of Rose Kushner's conclusions after interviewing thousands of women. Of patients whose breast cancer neither recurred nor metastasized—who were cured, in other words—Kushner noted that postmenopausal women, especially if widowed or divorced, seemed to react longer and more severely to mastectomy than younger married women.

Judy also discussed what Rose Kushner called "unrelated premastectomy psychological problems." Removal of the breast becomes a focus for unresolved dilemmas of marriage or other relationships, aging, attractiveness, loneliness. Judy mentioned one woman fighting a weight problem that had already hurt her love life before mastectomy happened.

I recalled Julia Child's sensible approach: "We have such a breast fetish in this country that women are led to believe that they're absolutely useless without them. Sexuality is a matter of attitude, not equipment." Julia Child, a cookbook author who teaches cooking on TV, is a public personality who, like Betty Ford and Happy Rockefeller, had a chance to speak out about her affliction and bravely did so, believing it would counteract fear.

Judy, who has met or worked with numerous models and stars of film, television, and music, remarked, "I really feel angry at people who have had breast surgery but keep it hidden for twenty years. The closet mastectomy people. Here they've had a glorious opportunity to speak over the media not only of breast surgery but of the fact they're alive and well—and they haven't done it. They're cowards. These people who earn their living by sexuality will talk or write about their bed partners but not about their mastectomies. They could do so much to counteract people's fear of cancer. If I were a superstar, I'd urge all women to examine their breasts, to seek mammography, and know these things can be lived through."

Judy continued, "There's too much emphasis on breast surgery today. It makes women fearful. If a woman's breast disease has been cured, after five or ten years why make more of it than, say, TB or pneumonia? Nowadays people in this country do not fear TB because they know it can be cured, if treated early. And there's no epidemic of it."

In the last century, TB was debilitating, pervasive, and if untreated, invasive from the lungs to other portions of a person's anatomy. Indeed, when I looked up tuberculosis in an old (1951) medical dictionary, all the symptoms from which the English writing family, the Brontës, withered one by one, were described, followed by, "Prognosis: generally fatal." During a public talk Dr. Strax remarked, "When I was a medical student, we had wards full of TB. We looked at TB X rays all the time. We were sending people for cures of years at Saranac Lake. Today we hardly hear of TB."

Although the tuberculosis rate is higher among the poor in this country, the disease in general is considered understood and controllable by present standards of sanitation and medical care against infectious diseases. People still die of it (3,280 in 1976, with a further 32,105 ill with it), but few fear an epidemic—or a chest X ray. Cancer has succeeded TB's image as the "white plague" of the twentieth century.

And people like Judy know its reputation frightens women from seeking diagnosis, especially if they see mastectomy as the only and inevitable treatment.

Judy contended, "It's *not* heroic to have a breast taken off. It doesn't have to be a major trauma that takes years to recover from. A woman can survive with one breast just as well as with two. Honestly, I've had more problems controlling my weight than I had over mastectomy," she said. "My life is just the same. I want people not to be so fearful. If the worst thing that ever happens to me is having my breast removed, I'll consider myself lucky."

When I asked Judy what she knew of risk factors for breast cancer in her own case, she replied, "None in particular except we were a big meat-eating family. My breast cancer is a family first. Before it, I was totally asymptomatic except for a sudden abscess in the other breast, which cured all right."

Her present medical care involves visits to both a gynecologist and a surgeon twice yearly and to her internist for a physical once a year. She does not have mammography "because my breasts are small and my doctor believes he could feel any problems in time." According to the latest guidelines (Chapter 13), routine mammography is not recommended for women under fifty. And small, dense breasts do not X-ray as successfully as those with more fatty tissue. However, many doctors would consider Judy sufficiently high risk to warrant regular mammography.

At the end of the interview Judy surrendered our milk in a saucer to the waiting cats. She had already caught one happy feline warming itself against the coffee pot on a hot kitchen burner. "Get down from there—you'll burn your *tush!*" she warned while she answered Betsy's questions. One of the poodles had nestled itself into sleep around my back.

Whatever Judy's life brings, I doubt she will find much time to brood.

21 / Saving Mind and Life: New Counseling

Dr. O. Carl Simonton of Fort Worth, Texas, is a radiologist who has combined physical treatment with research on those patients who achieve impressive survival records ("patients who live in excess of two years past incurable diagnosis" instead of the predicted six to twelve months). Nor is this survival time a period of drugged invalidism—the epitome of indignity and vulnerability. "Approximately 80 percent remain fully employed and socially active despite an incurable diagnosis. The majority express having had little or no pain associated with disease and remarkably few side effects from conventional treatment." And these people already have widely metastasized disease.

But who are these "Superstars—capital S out of respect" as Dr. Simonton terms them?

"The patients are verbal, confrontive, at times scrappy, and generally receptive and highly creative people. If more than two of these exceptional patients are in a room together, the air is thick with the contention of their very prominent egos. They have been known to be hostile, compulsive, and demanding upon occasion; rarely are they docile or obsequious."

They are younger than most persons when confronted with the diagnosis of incurable cancer (average age forty-four), and educated (average 17.2 years of formal schooling). On a battery of tests they score high in freedom from rigidity and overconventionality of behavior, in ego strength, energy level, self-reliance, willingness to accept responsibility for their own physical and mental condition.

This last characteristic forms the key to Dr. Simonton's multifaceted approach to cancer counseling. He developed cancer himself at age seventeen. As a radiologist, he later treated lung cancer patients who had refused to stop smoking. He wondered why. He is now in private practice with another radiotherapist and a team of psychologists, including his wife, Stephanie Matthews-Simonton, at the Cancer Counseling and Research Center, Fort Worth. To the standard trio of surgery, radiation, and chemotherapy, they have added a program of counseling, meditation, and self-confrontation called imagery therapy.

Not everyone who enters Dr. Simonton's office desires such training. He admits, "Over half of them will not participate in any form of psychotherapy. They will not attend group therapy. They will not use the relaxation-visualization techniques. Many of them not only will not talk about it, or allow us to talk to their families about the psychological aspects of their disease, but they might even go back to their physician and ask to be referred to another doctor."

Besides patients with active disease from Texas and around the United States, Dr. Simonton's group also treats patients now free of disease except for "one of the real residuals of cancer, and that is *fear*. . . . It is interesting to note that before a person has cancer, he may have a tennis elbow that aches occasionally. However, once he has had cancer, that aching tennis elbow suddenly represents the fear of metastasis. . . . These patients need concrete techniques they can use to deal with aches and pains."

Dr. Simonton's program is really a form of self-hypnosis—helping the patient mobilize his or her own forces after individual or group coaching. It begins with an orientation session. The patient attends "with as many family members and close friends as he would like to bring. We explain our concept of disease, how mind interacts with body and how attitude plays a role. We teach them a technique which we call relaxation and visualization. You might call it biofeedback without a machine, meditation, autogenic training . . . where they are told to visualize their disease and visualize their body's own immune mechanisms (or we call them white blood cells to make it simple) acting on that disease, three times a day every day."

He recommends further instruction via cassette and weekly group sessions plus the book *The Will to Live* by Dr. Arnold Hutschnecker.

Susi Heins, a Californian, was in her twenties when she noticed a lump in her groin and received the diagnosis "lymphoblastic lymphoma, general and incurable." After treatment by Dr. Virginia Livingston and biofeedback-imagery training from Dr. Kenneth Pelletier, a San Francisco psychiatrist, repeated sonography has shown her internal organs to be normal and without cancerous nodes. She now jogs a mile a day "although for months I could barely walk the course."

Three times per day she relaxes. "I let all the tensions of the day seep right into the carpet. . . . In this pleasantly relaxed state I imagine my cancer as putty balls and the force that fights it as 'The Little Dwarfs of Cologne' from a German fairy tale [Ms. Heins is German by birth].

"In the old days in Cologne, at night the baker and cobbler and butcher and tailor would leave their work and go home. Then the little dwarfs would appear and finish their chores, so when the tradesmen came back to work in the morning, their task was done. Well, my dwarfs march in to the tune of Prokofiev's 'Peter and the Wolf.' They carry big, heavy garden tools and hatchets. They start fiercely chopping and hacking and cutting away at my nodes. They throw the pieces onto a shovel, through the liver and kidney into the waste system. Then the white blood cells go to work. . . . The whole session takes about twenty minutes."

She and her husband "are again enjoying the Sierras backpacking, cross country ski touring, and downhill skiing." Admittedly Susi Heins' youthful optimism and strength helped win her fight.

Contrast her experience with that of an older patient with lung cancer metastasized to the brain. No doubt he received the same incurable diagnosis as Ms. Heins. This depressed man quit work to spend his days watching television and the clock to make sure his wife gave him his pain medication on time. He assured Dr. Simonton he was meditating successfully.

Dr. Simonton asked him what his cancer looked like to him and he said, "It looks like a big black rat." When Simonton asked him what his treatment looked like (he was receiving chemotherapy in the form of little yellow pills), he replied, "They look like little yellow pills and they go into my bloodstream and they look like tiny pills." Simonton also asked what happened between the pills and the rat. He said, "Well, he's sick for a while, but he always gets better, and he bites me all the harder."

Among "those factors predisposing and perhaps most agreed upon as personality characteristics of cancer patients," Dr. Simonton includes

- A great tendency to hold resentment and marked inability to forgive
- Tendency toward self-pity
- Poor ability to develop and maintain meaningful long-term relationships
- Very poor self-image.

At a cancer conference Dr. Simonton said, "I believe one of the big underlying factors behind all of the more superficial personality characteristics is basic rejection. The patient usually feels that he has been rejected by either one or both of his parents and consequently develops the life history pattern that we so commonly see in the cancer patient."

He carefully probes what he calls "the belief system of the patient and of his physician. Most patients see themselves as victims of the disease and not as having participated in the development of it. They also can see almost nothing that they personally can do to help themselves get well. Or at least this is the belief system that most of my patients present to me. . . .

"Another strike against the patients occurs when the

physician's belief system parallels that of the initial belief system of the patient: that the disease comes from without, that it's synonymous with death, that the treatment is bad, and that the patient has little or nothing that he can do to fight the disease.

"We've all been taught very poor tools for dealing with life. We hold too much in. Failure is never allowed. Success is everything. We are afraid to live fully because we would have something too dear to lose."

To enroll cancer patients in their own struggle, to end the stress-depression cycle, Stephanie Simonton begins by differentiating responsibility from blame. "For some reason we have a conception of responsibility being the same as blame. This is one reason for our inability as a society to deal with the emotional aspects of our diseases. We feel if we accept responsibility, then we are to blame, should feel guilty, or have done something wrong. We try to get across the idea to the patient that it's just as if you were to deny your body food for too long. We know that you would eventually die. . . .

"We have emotional needs and if these are denied, life loses its meaning. We will begin to seek the end of our life. We stress not that they should feel guilty, but that they have emotional needs that are not being met."

One cancer patient and his wife participated in several three-day group sessions in Fort Worth. She wrote that the method "outdid all the encounter groups and sensitivity training sessions I have ever participated in." She felt the doctors and leaders "were successful because they cared." They asked questions like: What deep need in your life is not being fulfilled? In what ways has life lost meaning for you? Why do you want to die? Why do you need to have cancer? Can you give two good reasons why you should be alive two years from now?

In an indifferent environment such questions would destroy someone. In a carefully managed situation with relaxation methods available to control tension, they seem to function as a deterrent to depression, a goad to utilize one's powers instead of naively investing doctors or relatives with total responsibility for care, cure, or miracles.

Dr. Simonton continues to match these patients with others of similar age and disease who do not participate in order to see "whether we can change both the quality and quantity of the patient's survival time by influencing his attitude."

Like many therapies, the Simontons' cancer counseling (relaxation, visual imagery, goal setting, evaluating sources of tension) succeeds with motivated, indeed self-selected individuals. Psychiatrists and other physicians criticize Dr. Simonton for proceeding without enough controlled studies, for claiming that his method is the primary reason that some patients live longer. One psychiatrist said to me, "It's akin to faith healing, and he is claiming to cure cancer."

Nevertheless, the Simontons' program has received sufficient notice for them to travel around the United States and train therapists. Their basic counseling program involves a weekend session of guided therapy. It is open to cancer patients as well as social workers and other professionals.

Journal Keeping

Harriet Wrye is a researcher in social and clinical psychology at Wright Institute, Los Angeles. For some years she has studied the belief systems of cancer patients, specifically through a project of tests, interviews, and journal-writing workshops for breast cancer patients. She is studying women who are at least one year beyond mastectomy.

In response to a question relating cancer to personality, she said, "We don't have data that can show the cause of cancer in the personality per se. We no longer think of a simple cause-effect relationship but of the mind and body as a unit—input on any level affects all levels. This is a systems, a feedback loop, idea rather than a cause-effect relationship. It's different even from the psychosomatic mind-body duality written about in the forties and fifties. That approach still posited *two* separate units, the mind and the body, interacting.

"With repeated stress—unsolved problems, feelings neither expressed nor otherwise brought to consciousness—the immune system can fail. In one sense, cancer may represent a body protective response gone awry the way pus formation around a wound is initially a healthy response of white blood cells to foreign bacterial invasion. If untreated, however, it can become a chronic infection, especially in a person whose immune response is poor through faulty diet, for example."

Did she believe there are people who can be considered "cancer-prone personalities"?

"The women I have interviewed don't exhibit one large recent loss so much as a pattern of fear and loss, of underlying insecurity, the sense that 'I'm not good enough.' "

"You mean, good enough at some task in the present—marriage or relating to a child?" I asked.

"No. A whole pattern of cumulative events begun in early life through contact with conditional love given by a parent who was immature. That is, if there is a past history of experiencing helplessness, lack of control, loss, or insecurity, breast cancer will reactivate these feelings. . . . Part of the healing process should be summoning one's *strengths.*"

There is a psychological test that inventories a woman's personal strengths to determine her typical patterns of responding to conflict, for instance. Harriet Wrye's investigation focuses on the relationship between an individual's beliefs about vulnerability and her efforts to find help within or outside herself.

One therapeutic tool to deal constructively with powerful emotion is journal writing, and Harriet Wrye has conducted journal workshops for recovered mastectomy patients. "I feel journal writing is so valuable for women who have had breast cancer. People are not accustomed to getting in touch with their inner selves. We do dialogues with important relationships, with sexuality, and with events. It's an inner journey." The aim of a journal-writing workshop is to share experiences and gain some concrete writing techniques which women can use later by themselves.

Harriet Wrye asks each woman to begin by choosing a symbol that represents herself or has personal meaning for her. After several attempts one woman remarked in frustration, "I can't think of anything but my children." Wrye added,

"And those children were already gone from home. One was in Europe."

She continued, "Some of the women realize they've been living in the future. A typical pattern would be, 'All my life I thought I'd have a chance to do whatever—travel, work maybe—after my children were grown, after an aged mother is gone, after my husband got the promotion. And now I've got breast cancer.' For such women, breast cancer provides both the opportunity and the need to transform their values, to change their relationships to life and people."

I asked about the differences between young and older women facing the cancer crisis. She replied, "Younger women seem more defensive. They are more denying of what is happening. By contrast, the older women I've interviewed are more anxious to make changes in their lives that they've never before made."

I asked Harriet Wrye's opinion of the notion that the "breast cancer personality" is a woman who has rejected some aspect of her sex role. Ms. Wrye answered, "Sex role is too broad a term. It could include everything in a woman's life. However, issues regarding separation and attachment are certainly sexual issues. Many women describe their own mothers as unresponsive, ambivalent, preoccupied, or having had no time for them as daughters. One woman asked, 'Why do I keep writing about my mother? She died years ago.' "

The women interviewed by Harriet Wrye reacted to, or compensated for, such mothering in two ways, either by not admitting or showing their own needs or by excessively devoting themselves to others' needs.

Dr. Simonton theorizes that his exceptional cancer patients (those with incurable diagnoses who lived at least twice as long as expected) are people who overcame the effects of inadequate parenting so that it did *not* become the touchstone for all subsequent loss and disappointment. "We wonder whether our exceptional patients emerged from this typical pattern with such impunity that they became totally self-reliant; whether they, in fact, substituted a belief in themselves in place of significant others to such an extent that their own integrity allowed them to overcome or stabilize incurable disease."

Becoming a Renewed Person

People who live poorly are people without a sense of mortality.
—BETTY ROLLIN

One topic this book pursues is the problem of who copes well with the devastating news of breast cancer and by what means. Tears? Talk? Faith in God? Supportive surgeon and friends?

A therapist I interviewed, recovered from breast cancer herself, believes women who cope best are those who have had, or pursue, breast reconstruction, doing what they can to restore their former physical selves. Other women, like Veronica (Chapter 18), cope by actively refusing mastectomy and arranging alternate effective care.

The key seems to be *active* response, for by agreeing to struggle against the disease (including the side effects of treatment), a woman seems to regain hope, her sense of normalcy.

Those who cope less well are those who do poorly with stress or setbacks in general, whose life history may fixate on one trauma, who expect existence to be easy, painless. Everybody has periods when negative feelings predominate—which is normal as long as they do not become a permanent response (or lack of response) to the problems that illness brings.

New approaches to cancer counseling help patients view the fight against illness as part of, not separate from, their life processes.

Dr. George Vaillant of Harvard Medical School wrote a book called *Adaptation to Life,* a longitudinal study that followed 268 Harvard graduates, including John F. Kennedy. A few sentences from a review of the book summarize the different functions of illness in one's life: "No one had been exempt from suffering; but *some* of the men responded to conflict and stress with ingenuity and creativity." Other subjects were "locked in childish or self-defeating patterns." One is projection, which is attributing to others "feelings of aggression that he could not acknowledge within himself."

The most successful became "aggressive in the service

of others. . . . The mature adaptive mechanisms enable a man to change something as unmarketable as despair into a commodity that others can cherish."

Regarding illness and connectedness with the human community: "While none of the men using mature ego defenses had recently been in poor health, as ascertained by objective medical examination, 36 percent of the men whose adaptive mechanisms were 'immature' were relatively unwell." And comparing friendly with lonely men: "Only 4 percent of the Friendlies were suffering from a chronic illness by the age of 52. Among the Lonelies, 47 percent had a serious physical ailment by that age."

New Hospital-Associated Programs

Dr. Eugene Thiessen, a Manhattan breast surgeon (Chapter 15), began and has continued sessions with one post-mastectomy counseling group at the Strang Clinic. Lee Miller, co-leader of this group, now called S.H.A.R.E. (for *Self-Help Action Rap Experience*), told me in early 1978 it had inspired the formation of two more active groups. "We discuss mutual problems following surgery and other cancer treatment. We are also working to end discrimination against cancer patients in jobs and in getting medical insurance." The group blends new mastectomy patients with those many years past surgery.

Lee Miller was planning a hot line information service to answer calls about breast cancer research, diagnosis, and treatment. Such a service should help the woman who finds a lump and needs more information *before* committing herself to pressures of any particular approach, even her gynecologist's examination.

Peggy D. (Chapter 3) attended a support group called TOUCH sponsored by the New Haven, Connecticut, Metro Unit. The meetings (biweekly for ten weeks), she said, "helped by allowing me to share with other cancer patients my concerns and to hear from their experiences that what was happening to me was not unique. . . . Talking with others in a similar situation, people who are six months or a year ahead of me in treatment or recovery, is great therapy. They have seen me grow from a nervous Nellie to a more secure person."

Considering that cancer strikes an estimated one of every four people in this country, learning ways to cope with the feelings aroused by it and by subsequent medical care should be a primary goal of community psychiatric service. Many group programs, however, have begun only recently on a tentative basis. They await further funding and personnel for larger-scale use. Make Today Count, begun by cancer patient Orville Kelly of Burlington, Iowa, in 1974, now has seventy chapters and over 3,500 members. It is the most widespread program to help families cope with terror, improve the quality of life, and combat prejudice against cancer patients.

The National Cancer Institute has funded several demonstration projects to study the psychological aspects of breast cancer over the course of the disease up to eighteen months postmastectomy. Each project stressed a different aspect— community education, developing a booklet, physician education, and crisis counseling of women and their families. At Montefiore Hospital in the Bronx I talked with Dr. Jimmie Holland, a psychiatrist and director of the Psychosocial Research in Cancer Group, and Joan Fromewick, a medical social worker.

The aim of this project was to identify the significant stresses at each stage of the disease plus the range of methods used to cope. In addition, the project provided continuous psychological support to normal women and their families. Patients ranged in age from thirty to seventy.

At Montefiore, each breast cancer patient who entered the study received an interview, psychological testing, and group counseling. Some of Dr. Holland's conclusions are:

Women with breast cancer had significantly higher anxiety levels than both psychiatric patients, and patients with coronary disease or other neoplasms [tumors]. . . . Women with any breast lesions score much higher . . . on death anxiety, mutilation, diffuse and overall anxiety. . . . The women who received these services [of the project] functioned better, are better adjusted, have less anger, less anxiety. . . .

A centralized team approach to Montefiore's cancer care reduces or avoids the fragmentation of services. A medical social worker handles support services, especially for the chronically ill. She arranges visiting nurse home care, financial assistance, group and individual counseling. For chemotherapy patients, a nurse-oncologist handles injections during home visits, changes dressings, takes blood and urine samples, and acts as liaison between patient and doctor. The patient advocate, a Reach to Recovery volunteer with counseling training, handles further breast cancer care, such as information on prostheses and help with insurance forms. Spanish-speaking staff are important to all aspects of treatment at Montefiore.

Dr. Holland stressed, "Our program increases the quality of life. We don't claim to prolong life or cure anybody. That's a function of physical, medical factors."

Joan Fromewick entered the staff lounge carrying a pair of crutches she had lent a patient, who had now happily returned them. The patient's bone fracture, healing well, was *not* due to metastasis; joy was evident on Ms. Fromewick's face.

We spent some time discussing the counseling and support work. "We can utilize community services patients don't know about. When patients are afraid to call the doctor, they can call us. We arrange the patient's medical schedule into a coordinated series of visits. We evaluate which symptoms need help and which don't require a physician's help.

"We give them permission to be angry, depressed, in shock. 'If your family can't handle it, talk to us.'

"Our different personalities on the staff are a plus factor. My strength is counseling patients and arranging practical details of their life support system. Questions on chemotherapy we can refer to Dr. Holland [whose husband, Dr. James Holland, of Mt. Sinai Medical Center, coordinates several national chemotherapy studies].

"It's good to have a staff *group*. We can talk about our own feelings, like depression and being afraid to hope. Watching people get better, watching people die—if we can't cure people, does that mean we can't do anything?" she asked suddenly.

She described postmastectomy patients in her groups as "open with their feelings. . . . We do not insist that people allow us into their system. We tell them about everything. They accept what they need.

"And doctors realize we are helping *them*. We are taking this patient's anxiety so she will be more together for the doctor." Nevertheless, Ms. Fromewick admitted obstacles. "Doctors who are opposed say things like, 'This lady is all put together. She doesn't need it,' or 'This other lady is too upset. Counseling would just upset her more.' "

One doctor whom Fromewick described as "very opposed to the program" seriously told a questioning husband, "Your wife is worried about her sexual attractiveness following mastectomy? Throw her on the bed and rape her. She'll *know* she's attractive."

Roberta Klein is a medical social worker at Sloan-Kettering Cancer Center, Manhattan. At the Second National Conference on Breast Cancer in the early seventies she said, "We in social work needed a quicker, more effective method to help people. What can we who surround the patient do?" She listed several goals, both sensible and useful.

Help her to express her feelings. "Permit her the tears that accompany her depression and help her to master those feelings."

Help her to sort out the real from the unreal.

Don't give false reassurances. "The patient who expresses fear of rejection, of perhaps dying, does not wish to be stopped with statements like, 'Don't worry, everything will be all right.' "

Help her to anticipate the future.

Help the family to understand the patient's feelings and to express theirs. "A husband has an equal need to communicate his concerns, about whether he will lose a wife, how he should respond to her postsurgery, what new needs she will have that he can fulfill."

Help the patient to consider how and what to tell those significant other persons in her life. "Special consideration should be given to the teenaged girl in a family. She, like her mother, has breasts and must wonder whether she, in her own time, shall face the same crisis. Will she frighten her daughter if she tells the truth?"

Crisis counseling of cancer patients as a community service open to many, instead of the rich few, is a whole new field for psychiatry. It becomes crucial whenever surgeons do not—and relatives cannot—give the help needed. All patients hope for cure, but they also deserve *care*—continuing concern.

RECOVERING

22 / Mary: "The Business of Living"

"I was operated on thirty-one years ago when medical care was superb! Are you sure you want to talk with *me?*" The white-haired woman with the twinkling blue eyes swept me into the sitting room of her cool, elegant apartment on Manhattan's Upper East Side.

"Of course," I answered. "You're exactly the person I'd like to interview."

We sat down on her beige sofa before a coffee table covered with letters, announcements, and graduation and other photos of grandchildren. Among the items on the wall hung a certificate of appreciation from the American Cancer Society for Mary's decades of service as a Reach to Recovery volunteer who now coordinates the work of some sixty volunteers visiting thirty-five hospitals in the New York City Division of ACS. With Terese Lasser, Mary helped found the Reach to Recovery program to aid postmastectomy patients.

While I was there, one granddaughter phoned from California with news of job and law school. Mary is reaping the fruits of a long life of joyful spirit and continuing involvement with others.

"How old do you think I am?" she asked.

"Well . . ." I hesitated. "The Cancer Society told me you're about eighty?"

"I'm *exactly* eighty. This year. On my eightieth birthday I offered to resign as head of Manhattan volunteers, but you know what they did? They gave me a birthday party instead." Mary smiled. "I work every day." She visits three hospitals near her apartment where surgeons have requested a Reach to Recovery volunteer.

We returned to the topic of the interview. "You know," Mary said, "my daughter had breast cancer, too. About six months before she died, she had a mastectomy. She didn't die of cancer but of complications related to cystinuria, a disease that causes kidney stones. When she was twenty-one, she had a kidney removed. They told her never to have children, but she had three beautiful babies. She was forty-five when she died." Mary's two sons, one of whom she calls "kid," are now about fifty.

Mary herself has participated in cancer research through donating blood samples for work in immunotherapy and urine for work in biological markers at Manhattan hospitals. Mary's interest in medicine began early. Trained as a bacteriologist, she worked at the University of Pennsylvania Hospital performing laboratory tests and reporting on results.

Like many women, Mary discovered the tumor in her left breast accidentally while in the bathtub. "It was the size of my little fingernail." At the time, she had finished menopause during which she had received hormones to stem heavy bleeding and clotting. She also had fibroid tumors, common and benign growths in or on the uterus, that had regressed due to menopause by the time she felt the breast lump.

She quickly saw "a family friend, who's an excellent surgeon," telling him, "I want this out right away." When her husband pleaded with her to obtain a second opinion or alternative to surgery, she countered, "I can't imagine being referred to a top-class man like him and not taking his opinion. If you spend a half hour in his office, you can tell by how he answers your questions how knowledgeable or competent he is. Right?"

I wondered whether doctors in the 1940s simply had more time, or *spent* more time answering family's or patients' questions. Mary added, "In my opinion, one of the smartest things a family can do is to get a doctor who's also a family friend and can evaluate new symptoms on the basis of a total history."

Although Mary signed the combined permission form allowing simultaneous biopsy and mastectomy if needed, she had her operation in two stages because of a problem known as the "false negative." The frozen section analysis of her tumor, done during surgery by the pathology lab, seemed negative for cancer, but a paraffin section ordered later by her doctor proved positive. Mary's kind of tumor, carcinoma *in situ,* has a favorable prognosis. Cancer that remains encapsulated in normal tissue, it has not spread beyond the breast nor has it involved the lymph nodes of the armpit. Mary's long life is also directly related to her early discovery of the tumor.

However, she was not informed of the pathology results for seven years—which was standard medical practice of the 1940s with cancer patients.

"So how did your doctor justify removing your breast and chest muscles and cutting into your underarm if he didn't say you had cancer?" I asked.

"He said he did it for precautionary reasons. And for seven years I didn't know I had cancer. My husband knew from the start. The doctor told me only when Mrs. Lasser and I started Reach to Recovery, and I asked him to refer patients to us."

"Weren't you angry at being deceived?"

"Of course. But remember this was the 1940s. By contrast, nowadays they read you the kiss of death as soon as you come from the operating room. Is that so much better?" Then she laughed. "Besides, while I was home recovering, I swam and played golf. In fact, just three months after the surgery, I beat that doctor at a game of golf. He was a lousy golfer!"

She sobered. "Of course, I had a husband plus three children to finish raising. When I left the hospital after five days—unbelievable then—it was Easter vacation. My teenagers were all home. The kids were sweet and noisy. I just went into my bedroom when it got too much. When I left the hospital, I had no time to feel sorry for myself. I went about the business of living.

"Well, I came home too soon. I filled up with fluid under the collarbone and had to return every other day for six weeks for needle aspiration of the fluid." A Hemovac drain apparatus connected immediately after surgery helps contemporary women minimize this painful fluid-retention problem. Mary slipped off the long paisley sleeve of her caftan and showed me part of the incision. Neatly done, it had healed well. Her left forearm, however, remains swollen—after three decades. No wonder Drs. George Crile, Sr. and Jr., and cancer patients themselves have attacked such debilitating and disfiguring surgery in women whose cancer is already far advanced or in women like Mary whose minimal cancer has a good prognosis.

Since Mary is left-handed, I wondered whether the arm pained her at night. She replied, "No," and recalled, "I had confidence in my doctor. I didn't know anybody who ever had breast cancer—no cancer in my family. My mother died at sixty-five of a heart attack. My doctor and my husband comforted me. I never felt sorry for myself. I'm lucky. . . . But when I did find out years later that I'd had cancer, I called that doctor a son of a bitch. Then we kissed and made up. He's eighty-two now and retired. We're still good friends."

She continued, "For years afterward when I had checkups I was scared they would find something. Now I have a twice-yearly checkup plus mammography once a year. I always say to them, 'Give me a good feel, please.'"

How did Mary's husband and teenagers react later in the postoperative period? "Well, they all knew I'd had my breast removed. However, regarding my husband I did the most awful thing when I came home. We used to undress together in our bedroom. For the first month I hid in the bathroom to undress. Naturally he thought I was rejecting him. Now I advise patients I see: don't make any unnecessary hurdles you then have to take down.

"I don't remember mourning loss of a breast per se, that is, my body image. However, those foam rubber pads, the ancestors of the good, weighted protheses they have now, never stayed in place, and I didn't have sense enough to anchor them with elastic. My husband and I arranged a signal system. Every time he rubbed his left ear, it meant, pull your bra down. It meant I was riding high on one side, was misplaced somehow." Because her breasts are ample, this problem caused her repeated discomfort that a smaller woman might not experience.

I asked about Mary's adventures as both a Reach to Recovery volunteer and a director of volunteer services. Each volunteer is a woman who has recovered successfully from a mastectomy herself—except in isolated geographical areas where a nurse or other trained woman can help. She brings to new patients exercise equipment, a lightly padded bra, a booklet, and individualized answers to questions.

Mary's postmastectomy advice is: "Postpone that first look at the incision until the doctor has removed both the bandages *and* the stitches." The flesh, while still swollen and tender, is flatter then, not trussed up by sutures. To a woman with a good marriage, she recommends asking the husband to share the first look. "I say, 'You have to take the initiative because your husband may be firghtened, too. Just say something like, "I'm scared to death to look at this. Will you help me?" ' "

Mary herself is a widow. When I inquired how she could assess the marriage of a woman she's never met before and a man she's never met at all, she replied, "I look at the photos on her bed table. I watch her reactions carefully, whether the tears well up. After a few minutes I may talk about her marriage in terms of *going home*. Going home may include neighbors who bake a cake and deliver it while they check which side her surgery is on. But it also includes readjusting to her normal sexual life, changing her self-image, and facing herself with one breast."

On talking with children, Mary recommends, "Answer questions truthfully, but don't make a big deal of it. And don't lie. I scared my daughter," Mary admitted, "so she wanted both her breasts cut off as prevention." Like other women I interviewed (Rita, Chapter 5), Mary found her breast cancer experience visibly distressed her daughter more than her sons. But much depends on the individual child's personality. "Give the facts, but don't be morbid. And remember that children have a pretty short attention span," even for topics disconcerting to adults. She recalled an anecdote about one son's rushing into the master bedroom just as she and her husband finished dressing for Saturday dinner out. "Tell me everything you know about where babies come from," he demanded.

She answered, "Well, Daddy and I are leaving now, but tomorrow morning you and I can have a nice talk. All right?"

He zipped on to his other insoluble problem. "Okay, if you don't want to talk about that, then why did Columbia lose today?" He and his father were fans of opposing ball teams, Columbia and Penn.

Like other recovered cancer patients, Mary has found herself also doing out-of-hospital counseling. An acquaintance had invited her to meet a European couple who heard about her Reach to Recovery work with apparently little interest in such a conversation topic. Six months later the same invitation was repeated; Mary couldn't figure out why. Her acquaintance said, "Mrs. —— is waiting. She wants to talk with you." Mary said to me, "You know, after all my experience I still didn't guess what was coming." During those months the woman had had a mastectomy and in her own country had found no one she dared approach about recovery problems or breast forms. "Here I'd assumed either they hadn't heard me or Reach to Recovery embarrassed them."

Reach to Recovery volunteers are carefully selected and trained. "We inquire of both their surgeons and internists about factors like emotional stability and ability to work with people." Volunteers are also matched with patients in areas like age and marital status. Of her New York volunteers, Mary noted their "dedication, loyalty, and beauty. Two-thirds of them also have full-time jobs."

Mary has spoken to large audiences at schools for registered and practical nurses. A letter about such a talk lay on her coffee table.

Each volunteer comes at the request or with the permission of a new patient's attending surgeon although there are various ways of nudging surgeons into the program. In one Westchester hospital near New York City, a patient-service representative, whose sister had a mastectomy, told me she supplies recovery room nurses with Reach to Recovery request forms and some brief patient data covering topics like bra and dress size, marital status, etc. Nurses insert a request form into the chart of each mastectomized patient so it becomes the first item her surgeon sees when he opens her record.

Surgeons are increasingly cooperative about such one-time visits to their recovering patients. Many value such a useful adjunct to their own care in returning a woman to full functioning and normal appearance. Others, however, remain resistant. Mary recalled one incident that occurred after a talk she'd given to an amphitheater full of medical people. Encountering her afterward, a famous male breast surgeon remarked, "If I allowed your Reach to Recovery to see one of my patients, I'd feel I was abandoning her."

"Yes, Doctor, and you've never had one of your bosoms removed either."

Twenty-five years after her organization's founding, one famous New York hospital still does not allow the program unless the patient specifically asks for it, "and then not always." With another hospital, she noted, "We are making slow but sure headway."

To close the interview, I read Mary this quotation from Roberta Klein of the Social Services Department, Memorial Hospital for Cancer and Allied Diseases, Manhattan:

That patient who successfully achieves these tasks [works through problems of the crisis period] must necessarily test strengths never before needed and perceive facts of herself never before apparent. Surely she can never be the same again; she is a stronger, prouder, more self-assured woman who has not only attained equilibrium but has grown.

Mary laughed. "Well, this psychological lingo wasn't in existence thirty years ago, but I'll forgive you. . . . I don't approve of people talking social service jargon when they haven't had the experience themselves except for having two bosoms, but I think that's a beautiful quotation.

"Finally, though, the chief person who can help a patient is herself. We all want crutches and maybe we all need them for certain periods to get better. But I believe people should use what God has given them inside themselves."

23 / *Physical Rehabilitation*

It took me a long time to get a good-fitting prosthesis and bra—and there are too few sympathetic fitters. —LORETTA, age forty

To gather material for this chapter, in addition to my interview with Mary (Chapter 22) I questioned Terese Lasser about Reach to Recovery, visited a postmastectomy boutique, and solicited opinions about breast reconstruction (plastic surgery) and some exercise programs.

Reach to Recovery

Reach to Recovery was begun in the mid-fifties after Terese Lasser's own radical mastectomy. Like many women, she found herself unprepared for the shock and mutilation of surgery and the unknowns of aftercare. She wrote:

I checked into the hospital expecting surgery so minor that I made no mention of it to my husband. . . . He thought I was playing in a golf tournament at the moment I was being wheeled into the operating room. . . .

I could not even grope for answers to the dreadful questions forming in my mind. I had never known anyone who had had a breast removed. That I, personally, could experience such a thing was simply inconceivable.

When she inquired about postoperative therapy, she was told:

. . . exercise of any kind . . . no guidance really. No actual supervision . . . to make a woman's comeback to her former way of life a challenging project rather than an ordeal of trial and error, distress and heartache.

In 1969 the Reach to Recovery program was merged into the American Cancer Society. By 1977, Reach to Recovery had over 10,000 volunteers in the United States and abroad. These are women like Mary, Judy, and Rita who have successfully readjusted after surgery and are able to help others with questions about prostheses, clothing, exercise, family and sexual life. The program now reaches about 50,000 (an estimated 67 percent) of the approximately 80,000 women who undergo mastectomy yearly. It has expanded to include male volunteers, and a Husband to Husband program that features a taped discussion by two men on topics related to cancer and family life. This approach provides needed help for husbands and wives who have cultural taboos against speaking about sexual matters.

At the request of attending surgeons, Rita, who is a Reach to Recovery volunteer, visits women her own age or older. In our interview she recalled one family situation where she helped avert a family crisis over mastectomy. A Latin American woman, unused to discussing sexual matters with her husband, had told him she was entering the hospital to have her cardiac pacemaker adjusted. Now she worried how to tell him the truth, fearing not that he would leave her but that the shock would make him get drunk and tell the whole family. When the wife suggested another man might speak with him, Rita found a willing male volunteer. The idea worked well, and Rita later helped the woman choose a prosthesis.

Terese Lasser told me, "We endorse and sell nothing. We only supply information. We try to ease everything we can for the patient. We help her talk, and we listen."

I asked Terese Lasser what changes the women's movement has brought in helping patients to request a Reach to Recovery visit. (The official request, however, must still come from the attending surgeon.) Mrs. Lasser estimated, "Three-quarters of patients have different attitudes now about discussing cancer or matters of feminine modesty."

Yet traditional attitudes about female roles and possibilities affect women of all ages. Terese Lasser continued, "I sat on the floor and rocked in my arms an eighteen-year-old girl from southern Europe because, unmarried and unpregnant as she was, she was still distraught that she wouldn't be able to *breast-feed* when the time came."

Mrs. Lasser travels widely on speaking tours despite one doctor's regular cautions. As I left, she remarked, "My doctor has been frightening me for thirty years. I just switched to another doctor."

Reach to Recovery has been criticized for being too prosthesis-oriented and for the fact that some visits, when done by an inappropriate volunteer, depress or bewilder rather than cheer the recipient. Volunteers themselves in some regions are stymied by doctors' releasing mastectomees after three, instead of five, days or longer in the hospital. This necessitates a home visit, which may not be as satisfactory for either volunteer or mastectomee.

However, for an immediate program of what amounts to crisis counseling of normal women on a range of topics— physical exercises and equipment, suggestions for hand and arm care, answers to nonmedical questions, help with prosthesis and clothing selection, revelation to husband, family, and neighbors, and reorientation to active living—there remains no program like it. It is also offered free to the patient, in contrast to some private therapies.

Patricia Lafferty, R.N., is Patient Service Representative at White Plains Hospital, White Plains, New York. Besides doing Reach to Recovery counseling, she has devised a repertoire of techniques to encourage surgeons to accept Reach to Recovery for their patients, such as getting the request form into the front of each new mastectomee's chart, and doing basic education of doctors on female viewpoints, such as the immediate need for a prosthesis in the form of the temporary bra Reach to Recovery offers. She told me how she convinced one doctor. "I made up a story about a lady who didn't want the whole neighborhood to greet her minus a breast or bra. Then I asked, 'If that were *your* wife, would you want this to happen?' "

Mrs. Lafferty would like to see nurses, instead of surgeons, allowed to present Reach to Recovery to the patient and to request it, if desired, as a routine part of postoperative nursing care.

Sometimes the patient herself, not the doctor, is recalcitrant about a visit. "One patient told the doctor to get out when she saw the scar for the first time, and he tried to explain Reach to Recovery."

Nurse Lafferty and I discussed the consent-to-surgery forms that loom so ominously over any woman entering for a biopsy. Legally a patient may consider or reconsider until administration of the preoperative drugs about forty minutes before surgery. If a patient in tears over her consent to a mastectomy changes her mind the day before, Mrs. Lafferty will enter her room carrying the signed form, and rip it up before the patient's eyes. She then leaves the pieces, promising the patient that she herself can decide whether or not to return the form to the nurse.

Postmastectomy Fashions

My mother turned a negative happening into a positive vehicle for herself. —ROB BLASHEK, age twenty-two, law student

After Joni Blashek had a mastectomy over a decade ago, she sold prostheses for some time until she realized, "To my knowledge there were and are very few, if any, street-level boutiques catering to women who have mastectomy." She finally opened a store called Natural Look in White Plains, New York, to help meet the needs of suburban women. She offers sympathy, combined with expert fitting advice, and a wider range of prostheses and fashions than a woman usually finds in a bra shop or department store.

No one claims that a few ounces of silicone or foam rubber can ever replace a breast or help somebody live with the fact of cancer. Prostheses are devices that help women look normal in fashions that, for better or worse, still require a symmetrical bosom.

Reach to Recovery maintains an updated list of manufacturers of quality prostheses of different materials, as well as swimsuits, daytime and nighttime bras, nightgowns, and blouses, plus the names of stores that stock these items.

Regenesis is one such shop. Based in Manhattan, it sends its catalog to a mailing list of 10,000 people in the United States, Europe, and Latin America. Its selection ranges from bathing suits, beach dresses, and blouses through underwear, nightgowns, and evening gowns. Prostheses of several kinds are available and range in price (1978) from $50 to $150, depending on size and filler. A woman's needs, measurements, and preferences are kept on file so that future mail orders are possible.

On the windowsill facing the Regenesis store entrance is a foot-high bronze statue of a god/goddess with one breast—and three eyes and four arms—named Ardhanishiva. One of the many manifestations of the Hindu god Shiva, it was brought from the East by Chandra, a Regenesis employee. It represents one of Shiva's androgynous forms uniting male and female energies. When I had learned its name, the saleslady remarked of its one-breastedness, "Nobody would look like that without special help from God!"

Breast Reconstruction

If you are a woman who has had a mastectomy, no doubt you wonder about the possibility of breast reconstruction. Dr. Reuven K. Snyderman, Clinical Professor of Plastic Surgery at Rutgers Medical School, Greenbrook, New Jersey, has a general practice in plastic surgery, and breast implants and reconstruction have beome one of his specialties. From two or three implants per year a decade ago, he now does two or three per week.

I met him while we both participated in a breast cancer discussion, videotaped for television, in Princeton, New Jersey. He showed slides of typical reconstructive work, including a close view sent by a young woman clothed in a smile, a tan—and a multicolored bikini. Neither scars nor indentations from her standard radical surgery were visible, and Dr. Snyderman had helped achieve the rest—a renewed breast that rose beautifully above her suit top, matched, to the eyes of the average observer, with the remaining breast. Clothed views of other women in bras, slips, even a tight tee shirt seemed so normal-looking that one forgot to wonder, "Which breast was it?"

"Breast reconstruction isn't new," Dr. Snyderman explained. "What is new is that there's now an easier method—silicone implant. And breast surgeons are doing less disfiguring operations—modified radical instead of standard radical surgery."

For a woman with a good base of skin over the chest wall, Dr. Snyderman completes implantation and reconstruction in a one-stage procedure. Some breast surgeons are now doing mastectomy with a horizontal incision that follows the skin's natural tension lines and is easier to repair. One woman I heard of agreed to a mastectomy on the condition that a plastic surgeon enter the operating room to advise her surgeon on the placement of the incision and to handle the suturing—all to facilitate later reconstruction. Another woman had the breast removed, keeping, however, as much as possible of the breast skin in place. This skin, alive and well, was sutured, awaiting reconstruction. When a resourceful woman meets a negotiable surgeon, a variety of medically safe compromises becomes possible.

Silicone implants are round transparent bags in various sizes prefilled with silicone gel that looks and feels like "heavy water." Some surgeons insert the basic bag or envelope, then inflate it with gel or saline solution. Dr. Snyderman prefers the prefilled, presealed, internal prosthesis to avoid the danger of leakage. The process involves implantation of an inert object; it does not involve injection of a substance, like liquid silicone.

Dr. Snyderman waits at least six months postmastectomy "until the skin on the chest wall moves freely," indicating the flaps of the mastectomy incision have healed. Some surgeons advise a longer wait if a woman has had invasive cancer (instead of carcinoma *in situ*) and/or a recurrence in the same breast area seems likely. Eighty percent of recurrences happen within three years of the first surgery.

A woman arrives in the operating room wearing her usual bra and external prosthesis. On her skin Dr. Snyderman draws the underwear outline to gauge placement of the implant so it—and the new incision—will fall inside the bra line, approximately equal with the other breast. After she is anesthetized, he makes the new 6-centimeter (about 2½-inch) incision at the base of what will be the reconstructed breast. He does not reopen the mastectomy incision because scar tissue is not sufficiently elastic and he does not want to jeopardize its blood supply. He then inserts the silicone implant (transparent bag) of appropriate size. The operation is simplest for a small-breasted woman needing minimal silicone and resultant stretching of skin over it. A larger woman may also need the remaining breast reduced in size via incisions beneath it and around the nipple to attain more evenly matched results. If a woman desires an areola (dark skin, somewhat raised to simulate a nipple) on the new breast, it can be grafted from the areola of the other breast.

Depending on the procedures needed or wanted, the surgery requires forty-five minutes to two and a half hours. A woman averages five days in the hospital.

I must add that such surgery, indeed any further hospitalization, is not for every woman who has already endured the stresses of mastectomy, cancer, perhaps irradiation. Three mastectomees participating in our videotaped discussion said they were curious about reconstruction but would not seek it for themselves. However, in the summer when an external prosthesis can be annoying, one said she was tempted. Dr. Snyderman termed the surgery "one more modality to help a patient return to normal life."

The woman who desires breast reconstruction may do so for a number of reasons. Women dissatisfied with an external prosthesis which may cause constant discomfort are most eager for the internal alternative. Dr. Snyderman mentioned an airline stewardess whose external prosthesis shifted position every time she leaned over to offer food and drinks. There are also mastectomees who have never achieved a correctly weighted prosthesis and as a result suffer chronic neck-ache or backache.

Women wanting to resume their former easy wearing of leotards, bathing suits, or strapless sportswear also desire it. Elise remarked, "Happiness represents not having to take one out of the bra in order to stick it into the swimsuit." Many of Dr. Snyderman's reconstruction patients simply want to look normal in a nightgown or underwear.

Rose Kushner tells a story on herself illustrating that no matter how well a mastectomee adjusts to her postsurgical body, in this breast-oriented culture she retains a sense of difference, even of shame. On separate occasions in two American cities, fire alarms rang at night in a hotel and a motel where she was staying. As she arose from bed, her first action did not involve flinging a bathrobe over her nightgown. It was rather to dress completely beginning with bra and prosthesis, despite the alarm ringing, because "I'll never go down with only one." Both times she arrived in the lobby, she discovered she was the only person fully awake and dressed in street clothes. "And the second time it happened," she mused, "I even had an attractive nightie with a dacron puff inside it."

In my opinion, reconstructive surgery remains for the highly motivated. Since some insurance plans unfortunately define any plastic surgery as "elective" or "cosmetic," a woman may need to pay the entire hospital and surgical cost herself. To help ensure safe and aesthetic results, it is wise to seek a physician who is a board-certified plastic surgeon (diplomate of the American Board of Plastic Surgery). This means that he or she has done a specialized residency in plastic surgery (distinct from general surgery) in addition to the basic eight years of medical school. Your county medical society or the *Directory of Medical Specialists,* a reference book found in many libraries, gives the names of such board-certified plastic surgeons.

In 35 to 40 percent of patients who receive reconstruction, a fibrous capsule of normal tissue gradually encloses the implant, making the breast firmer to the touch than the other one. Palpation and mammography are more difficult but not impossible, although opinions on this differ.

And how does reconstruction look? The slides I saw

showed patients, young and older, before and after. Minus clothes, the results were certainly better than the washboard or even concave appearance that radical mastectomy can cause. However, without skin grafting, a vertical or transverse mastectomy scar, elevated through reconstruction, seemed *more* noticeable. And like other surgery, breast reconstruction remains an art, never an exact science. A perfect match is not guaranteed. Reconstruction does restore a woman's cleavage so that, when clothed, she looks and feels stylish again, but it cannot, of course, restore the physical function of the chest muscles or mammary tissue.

Dr. Snyderman honestly admits results in the nude are "no cosmetic triumph." Breast reconstruction's chief advantages involve looking good in underwear and clothing that no longer need special tailoring and the fact that an internal prosthesis, unlike the external apparatus, need not be replaced every few years—or remembered every morning. Dr. Snyderman has healthy patients still satisfied with a reconstruction done fifteen to twenty years ago.

I asked Dr. Snyderman his opinion of subcutaneous mastectomy, a procedure recommended by some surgeons for high-risk women needing repeated biopsies for benign disease. Scooped-out breast contents are replaced with a filler inside the remaining skin and nipple. "I condemn subcutaneous mastectomy. The reason is that I don't feel, in most hands, enough tissue is removed," Dr. Snyderman answered. "I believe in prophylactic mastectomy for these women." He defined this as removal of the breast, the tail of the breast, and a number of underarm lymph nodes (a bit short of a modified radical, in other words).

He mentioned one woman with a three-generational history of breast cancer who had already endured the ordeal of seven biopsies. All had proven benign. Nevertheless, she decided on prophylactic mastectomy of that breast, performed by another surgeon. (Plastic surgeons, of course, do not do biopsy or mastectomy.)

Prophylactic mastectomy removes the breast, usually leaving nodes and muscles. It amounts to what is called *total* (or *simple*) mastectomy. While the thought horrified some women I interviewed, others who consider benign disease a risk factor for malignancy in their cases saw such a mastectomy as adding considerably to their peace of mind. With all surgical procedures now under debate after nearly a century of standardized treatment, with doctors denigrating one another's research and results (not to mention personalities and patients), it would be cruel to belittle any choice on which a woman has staked her very life.

In *A New You,* another plastic surgeon, Dr. James O. Stallings, writes:

Most general surgeons feel that if they've cured a woman of cancer and the wound has healed, she should be grateful for being alive. But they do not consider the emotional blow which the operation has inflicted on her. It's not that they are unkind, but most general surgeons are men and they are just not oriented to understanding and empathizing with the importance of the breasts to a woman's feelings about herself. As a result, they are generally disinterested, skeptical, or downright opposed to what plastic surgery can offer their patients.

Dr. Snyderman remarked, "I get the questions other doctors should have answered." Conservative general and breast surgeons should see that if reconstruction is medically safe and will help a woman regain her former occupational, social, and sexual life, she should be helped to pursue it.

In July 1977, Francine Timothy, director of Reach to Recovery in Chicago, spoke in favor of breast reconstruction to 1,700 people at an American Cancer Society conference on human values and cancer. Mrs. Timothy stated, "Whether a woman can have breast reconstruction is entirely up to the surgeon, but she should at least be allowed to want one without being judged. Many women have no idea whom they could ask questions about a reconstruction, and often don't ask any at all out of timidity. It is the fear of being judged vain or frivolous that keeps some women from looking into the possibilities."

She related an incident involving a woman facing the loss of one breast. When her surgeon asked how old she was, she said, "Fifty-two." He replied, "Then why do you care? You're not going to seduce anyone." This is the attitude described by Natalia (Chapter 12)—that any woman who expresses more than minimal regret over losing a breast or, worse yet, insists on keeping it must be promiscuous or otherwise deranged.

Mrs. Timothy stressed that while women of all ages and personality types "care desperately about being obliged to live with only one breast, perhaps reconstruction is almost more important to an older woman. A mastectomy is particularly hard on a woman who is already having trouble accepting the fact of growing older."

Physiotherapy

I spoke with a physiotherapist, Susan Greenberg, of New York Hospital, whose clinic helps postmastectomy patients with severe swelling or frozen muscle problems. "With radical mastectomy, a lot of women get lymphedema [swelling]. A lot of women become afraid to use the arm," she said. "We try to strengthen the arm, including its range." Ms. Greenberg combines exercises with deep breathing, relaxation, and massage. A physiotherapist is trained in careful evaluation of symptoms to choose the right combination of treatment.

For difficult breast cases, a Jobst compression unit exists. This is a machine on wheels designed to augment circulation in the arm—an electrical version of the surgical elastic sleeve. The patient dons a plastic sleeve, elevates her arm, squeezes her hand into a fist while the machine pumps rhythmically along the arm toward the heart.

Ms. Greenberg's work also includes home visits to some postsurgical patients until acute symptoms subside. "Most insurance policies will cover physiotherapy in the home, which most people don't know," Ms. Greenberg told me.

When Veronica Gardos returned with a swollen and frozen shoulder after a combination of business, travel, and incorrect physiotherapy in Australia, Ms. Greenberg's daily hour of physiotherapy at Veronica's apartment helped restore movement to her right arm and side.

Rita, by contrast, still has soreness in her arm and

shoulder. "They tell you it will last only a few months, but it's much longer than that. Years. Even now I know there are things I can't do. Or if I do them, I pay for it in soreness and stiffness. My arm remains slightly swollen all the time."

The Encore Program

For women who lack money and opportunity to dream of either breast reconstruction or private physiotherapy or psychological counseling, since the sixties the YWCA has pioneered a low-cost program called Encore. It combines rhythmic exercise, swimming, clothing advice, and rap sessions to help mastectomees.

Begun by a nurse, Helen Glines Kohut, herself a mastectomee, it was pilot-tested in twenty-four YWCAs throughout the United States. Sessions of 1½ hours per week are open to women as early as three weeks after surgery. Medical permission is needed. Since not every community has a Y, a program for training Encore leaders is also available. This is designed to interest dance, exercise, or gym instructors in facilities beyond Y locations. Some yoga teachers, for example, hold classes in stretching and relaxation techniques for mastectomees.

Mrs. Kohut remarked of her program, "When these women first come to class, they're wrapped in a cocoon of fear and self-doubt. Gradually they emerge to value themselves as women again." She understands very well the courage it may take for a woman to come "out of the closet" and live life in her own community again.

24 / Mary Behr: Reforming Cancer Aftercare

"We are fast becoming a one-breasted society."

This is Mary Behr's conclusion based on the fact that, of some 91,000 American women who get breast cancer yearly, the majority will receive some version of radical mastectomy—and begin to experience the financial, emotional, and job-related discrimination that afflicts any cancer patient who does not attempt to hide what has happened.

In 1976, four years after her radical mastectomy, Mary Behr succeeded in getting the New York State legislature to exempt from state and local taxation all orthopedic devices—some 350 items—bought by the handicapped in the state. Prostheses and bras for mastectomees, wheelchairs, custom-made limbs, walkers, crutches, bandages, bedpans, and hypodermic syringes for diabetics are a few. Also included are eyeglasses and hearing aids. By Governor Carey's estimate, the total saving to the handicapped is over $12 million annually—$7 million in state taxes and $5.25 million in local taxes.

Mary is currently involved in exposing the pervasive discrimination against cancer patients. She would like to end denial of employment, health insurance that refuses to cover mastectomy by terming it "cosmetic surgery," and "anticancer insurance" that insures the family of someone recovered from or afflicted with cancer, but not his or her own life. Thus far hidden from widespread notice, all these are successful strategies to make or save money at cancer victims' expense.

One of Mary's letters went to Congressman L. H. Fountain of North Carolina, who chaired a 1977 House subcommittee investigation into federal cancer research, which now receives an $815 million annual budget. About $8.6 million of this is used for breast cancer grants awarded by the Breast Cancer Task Force of the NCI Division of Cancer Biology and Diagnosis.

Mary alerted Congressman Fountain to the multiple needs of breast cancer patients for moderately priced prostheses, trained fitters in cancer centers to advise on clothing problems, review boards to examine the quality of mastectomy surgery, "especially in smaller communities where women do not have access to the top hospitals and surgeons," and more mastectomees' participation in policy decisions and the use of funds by the American Cancer Society.

Mary works from her home in upstate New York. Her husband is public relations director of a community college. I naturally wondered whether her knowledge of political strategy had resulted from participation in the struggles of the sixties. She shook her head. "No. Not at all. This is the first time."

Mary's own bout with cancer began when she looked into the mirror and discovered a 1-inch lump in the upper part of one breast. It proved malignant. She was fifty-one years old at the time. Her husband and grown son became "the principal supports that helped me through this nightmare." Wanting to avoid the anxiety of a two-stage operation, she had biopsy and radical mastectomy combined. Radiation—twenty-three cobalt treatments—followed. She agreed to these procedures. "There was no other choice."

The surgery left no permanent swelling although the scarring, which extends to the outside of her upper arm, is disfiguring and humiliating to an active, stylish woman. "A woman's whole life depends on looking as good as she can." Mary described at length the pain of shopping for clothes, assisted by salespeople who are either noncaring or oversolicitous if she must explain why she can't wear some latest fashion, especially the sleeveless or off-the-shoulder outfits she once enjoyed. Of salespeople, she said, "They just don't understand."

When I asked how she dealt with negative emotions—fear, anger, mourning—she responded, "I got tired of having people tell me, 'We all must die' or I 'could have got killed by a car.' There is so much being done with cobalt and chemotherapy now, yet we are burying 1,100 cancer victims every day. Fear never leaves you. Anger—a woman told me her husband had a colostomy a year ago and six months later she had a radical mastectomy. Each night when they undress and look at each other's mutilated bodies, they cry at the sight.

"I am weary of hearing smooth talk that adds nothing to the real effort to find a preventative for cancer from people who are in a position to help get the government to give a top national priority to this search. Trying to pacify cancer victims with slogans, poetry, and philosophical utterances is a poor substitute for harnessing all the resources of science, research, and medicine to a preventative, which is our only real hope."

For two years after surgery, Mary paid the 7 percent New York State sales tax on her prosthesis and the related items she needed. However, it began to seem like "putting salt on the wounds."

"The more I thought about it, the angrier I got. It seems like such an inhumane way to tax people." From legislators, physicians, pharmacists, church groups, and others in her city, she gathered over 3,000 signatures on a petition requesting a change in the tax law. After talking with those in power in both houses of the state legislature, she achieved repeal of the tax in a year of financial crunch when others warned her not to expect any reform. When someone asked her who would compensate the state for the lost revenue, she replied, "Who will compensate *me* for the loss of my breast?"

In late 1977 she traveled to California to begin lobbying there. Hearing of her efforts, the American Orthopedic and Prosthetic Association (AOPA) agreed to lobby in Washington for national repeal of all sales taxes on orthopedic and prosthetic appliances.

Mary explained, "The millions of people who have

cancer have not been heard. The prominent people have been heard. The rest of us are just struggling day to day.

"The whole country has been lulled by promotions saying, 'You can lead a normal life. We are working for a cure.' There is no such thing. You finish treatments and you leave. You don't dare to complain or you are compared to someone they think is doing great. You live from day to day. Now everything is after the fact: after you get it.

"A cancer patient can't even die in dignity. By the time each last cell is worn away, you are a burden to your husband, your family financially. You have your own husband and children glad your own pain and theirs is over with.

"We get action from our legislators only when we show them our interest in a subject, and the interest in this case is a matter of saving our lives and the lives of our loved ones from this killer disease, which strikes rich and poor alike. I tell my friends, 'Don't bring a cake and macaroni salad to my house after I die. All it takes is a letter and a fifteen-cent stamp *now*' to the Senate Health Committee, chaired by Senator Ted Kennedy, or to your own congressman."

Her efforts at insurance reform began when she saw an ad, phoned an anticancer insurance company in Georgia, and discovered their annual sales to families of cancer patients, not to patients themselves, are $150 million. A typical premium is six dollars per month. She commented, "They won't insure the cancer patient herself, of course, because they might lose money on that. This is preying upon people's fear and guilt at having burdened their families with their own cancer cost and care."

An orthopedic supplier in Mary's city requested insurance payment for a prosthesis and related supplies. The insurance company rejected the claim. In their policy, mastectomy appeared as "cosmetic surgery," implying that it's elective. Mary protested, "Do you think women *choose* to have their breasts taken off?" The supplier changed insurance companies. The original company rewrote that section of its policy.

Mary Behr's own mother died of cancer at age forty-two. She gets angry whenever anyone ignores or underestimates the hardship—physical, financial, emotional—that cancer patients endure when they discover the disease and when they try to readjust to society. But she is determined to do whatever she can.

The
Future...

Do you think they will perform mastectomy forever or will they find
another way? —QUESTION TO TERESE LASSER

Like mastectomy, so much about breast cancer has seemed "forever," continuing cancer's reputation as something treated or suffered in silence, with dread. Yet as you have seen in this book, even the entrenched radical mastectomy is yielding to other treatments that save women's bodies and lives. And many researchers, not just nutritionists, now view—and therefore fight—cancer as a systemic disease. A decade ago both these ideas seemed radical rhetoric engaged in by only the few who dared to challenge prevailing wisdom.

If you discover a breast problem, seek responsible care. But choices about that care are, and should be, also in *your* hands. Accept what is good but, as Mary Behr and others have done, continue to question whatever seems wrong to you as a woman, a patient, and as a human being eager to live.

Help make "another way."

APPENDIXES

I / Cancer-Related Words

adjuvant—refers to treatment, such as chemotherapy or ir-radiation, added to a primary therapy, usually surgery.

age-adjusted rate (of death or disease incidence)—the number who die or contract a disease in each age interval expressed as a fraction of those alive at the beginning of the interval.

amino acids—chief chemical components of proteins, strung together like beads on a chain to form the principal constituents of cell protoplasm.

antibody—protein (immunoglobulin) formed by the body's immune system to react with foreign proteins or other large molecules.

antigen—any of various materials (microorganisms, foreign proteins, etc.) that after a latent period induces a state of sensitivity and/or resistance from the host through production of antibodies.

areola—pigmented area around the nipple.

axilla (adj., axillary)—armpit.

biological or biochemical marker—elevated amount of a body substance that might indicate presence of cancer or other physiological activity.

biopsy—removal of a portion of living tissue for examination.

capillary—minute blood vessel.

carcinoma—cancer of cells of skin, glands, or mucous membrane tissues or linings. A woman's breasts, together termed "the breast," are modified sweat glands. Three common infiltrating carcinomas in the breast are scirrhous (one-half of all breast cancer), exhibits hard nodules composed of columns of epithelial cells separated

227

by calcified fibrous tissue; *medullary,* large, soft tumor composed of dedifferentiated epithelial cells arranged in glandular formation; faster-growing but with better prognosis than scirrhous; *mucinous,* also called gelatinous, mucoid, colloid; has abundant mucin, grayish translucent substance secreted by dedifferentiated cells; slow-growing.

carcinoma in situ—a localized and curable form of cancer. Pathologic evidence shows cell changes of the type associated with invasive cancer but these have not extended to adjacent structures.

CEA—carcinoembryonic antigen; protein material isolated originally from colon cancer cells; appears useful for diagnosis and assessment of treatment.

comedo carcinoma—form of cancer in which plugs of dying malignant cells may be expressed from the ducts.

corticosteroids—corticoids; chemical substances produced by the outer portion of the adrenal gland.

crude rate (of death or disease incidence)—rate per unit of time per so many members of the population.

cytoplasm—substance of a cell, exclusive of nucleus; liquid material of a cell.

DNA—deoxyribonucleic acid; one of the two nucleic acids found in all cells. The other is RNA. They exert primary control over life processes in all organisms.

endocrinology—science of the internal secretions and their physiological and pathological relationships.

epidemiology—science of studying the groups of people who get a disease, their ages and other characteristics, and where it is most prevalent. In reference to cancer, it does not imply that the disease is contagious or infectious.

epithelium (adj., *epithelial*)—cellular layer covering all free inner and outer body surfaces, including glands, skin, mucous membrane linings. Carcinoma is cancer of epithelial cells.

estrogen—hormone formed by ovary, placenta, adrenal cortex in females; by testes in males; by some plants. Three of its components or *fractions* are estriol, estradiol, and estrone.

etiocholanolone—an end product of adrenocortical and male hormone use, found in urine of males and females.

etiology—the cause of a disease.

fibroadenoma—common benign solid tumor.

fibrocystic—refers to benign breast disease characterized by formation of sacs of liquid or semisolid material with a conspicuous amount of fibrous connective tissue.

gene—a unit of heredity; a segment of a cell's or virus's DNA which specifies synthesis of a particular protein.

histology—microscopic study of tissue structure, normal and pathologic.

hormone—chemical product of an endocrine gland which, when secreted into body fluids, has a specific effect on other organs.

hyperplasia—increase in number of cells in an organ or tissue, excluding tumor formation.

immunotherapy—treatment directed at rendering the human body relatively resistant to a certain disease.

lesion—wound, injury, pathologic change in tissues. Precancerous lesions are changes in tissue not yet malignant but definitely abnormal.

lumpectomy—excisional biopsy; removal of the lump plus a margin of surrounding tissue.

mammography—X-ray examination of the breast.

mastectomee—person who has had a breast removed.

mastectomy—surgical removal of a breast. Different types of this surgery are the *standard* Halsted *radical* that removes breast, chest muscles (pectoralis major and minor), lymph nodes in armpit. The *supraradical* removes the foregoing plus some rib sections plus nodes under the breastbone (internal mammary nodes) or above the collarbone (supraclavicular nodes). The *modified radical* removes the breast and armpit nodes but leaves chest muscles intact. The *simple* (or *total*) removes only the breast, including its extension into armpit fold. The *partial,* also called *wedge* or *segmental resection,* removes only a portion of the breast. The *subcutaneous* removes breast contents, leaving nipple and skin.

metastasis (adj., *metastasized*)—apperance of cancer in a part of the body remote from the primary tumor, via bloodstream or lymphatic system.

MTV—MuMTV; mouse tumor virus; causes breast cancer in some strains of mice.

node—one of numerous round, oval, or bean-shaped bodies that collect and transport lymph, the transparent fluid part of blood.

norepinephrine—a form of adrenal hormone. Amount is thought to be elevated during depression.

oncologist—cancer specialist, particularly in chemotherapy.

oophorectomy—ovariectomy; surgical removal of ovaries.

psychosomatic—pertaining to influence of mind or higher functions of brain (emotions, fears, desires) upon the body, especially in relation to disease.

recurrence—reappearance of cancer in the same organ or upon the surgical incision that removed the original malignancy; to be differentiated from *metastasis.*

sarcoma—cancer of a connective tissue, such as bone.

sonography—examination of the body or an organ via sound waves to produce an echogram image.

thermography—examination of the body or an organ via a temperature map made by infrared sensing devices.

tumor—abnormal mass of tissue, whether malignant or benign.

vaccine—suspension of attenuated or killed microorganisms administered for prevention, amelioration, or treatment of infectious diseases.

virus—disease agent, smaller than bacteria, that requires living cells to grow and reproduce.

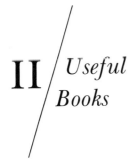

II / Useful Books

Cope, Oliver. *The Breast: Its Problems—Benign and Malignant—and How to Deal with Them.* Boston: Houghton Mifflin, 1977.

Crile, George. *What Every Woman Should Know About the Breast Cancer Controversy.* New York: Macmillan, 1973.

Cudmore, L. L. Larison. *The Center of Life, A Natural History of the Cell.* New York: Quadrangle Books, 1977.

East West Foundation. *A Dietary Approach to Cancer.* Boston, 1975.

Everson, T. C., and Cole, W. H. *Spontaneous Regression of Cancer.* Philadelphia: Saunders, 1966.

Fredericks, Carlton. *Breast Cancer: A Nutritional Approach.* New York: Grosset & Dunlap, 1977.

Germann, Donald. *The Anti-Cancer Diet.* New York: Wyden Books, 1977.

Gerson, Max. *A Cancer Therapy: Results of 50 Cases.* 1958. Available from Foundation for Alternative Cancer Therapies, New York.

Glasser, Ronald. *The Greatest Battle.* New York: Random House, 1976.

Hutschnecker, Arnold. *The Will to Live.* New York: Prentice Hall, 1966.

Kelley, William Donald. *One Answer to Cancer.* 1974. Available from Foundation for Alternative Cancer Therapies, New York.

Kushner, Rose. *Breast Cancer, A Personal History & an Investigative Report.* New York: Harcourt Brace Jovanovich, 1975.

Lasser, Terese. *Reach to Recovery.* New York: Simon & Schuster, 1972.

231

LeShan, Lawrence. *You Can Fight for Your Life, Emotional Factors in the Causation of Cancer.* New York: M. Evans, 1977.

Livingston, Virginia. *Cancer: A New Breakthrough.* Los Angeles: Nash Publishing Co., 1972.

Mae, Eydie. *Eydie Mae—How I Conquered Cancer Naturally.* San Diego: Production House, 1975.

Papaioannou, Anaxagoras. *The Etiology of Human Breast Cancer: Endocrinological, Genetic, Viral, Immunological, and Other Considerations.* New York: Springer-Verlag, 1974.

Pilgrim, Ira. *The Topic of Cancer.* New York: Crowell, 1974.

Seaman, Barbara, and Seaman, Gideon. *Women and the Crisis in Sex Hormones.* New York: Rawson Associates, 1977.

Seidman, Herbert. *Cancer of the Breast, Statistical and Epidemiological Data.* New York: American Cancer Society, 1972.

Selzer, Richard. *Mortal Lessons, Notes on the Art of Surgery.* New York: Simon & Schuster, 1976.

Simonton, O. Carl, and Simonton, Stephanie. *Getting Well Again.* Los Angeles: J. Tarcher, 1978.

Stallings, James O. *A New You, How Plastic Surgery Can Change Your Life.* New York: Mason/Charter, 1977.

Stoll, Basil. *Risk Factors in Breast Cancer.* Chicago: Yearbook Medical Publications, 1976.

Strax, Philip. *Early Detection.* New York: Harper, 1974.

Sutton, P. M. *The Nature of Cancer.* New York: Crowell, 1965.

Vaillant, George F. *Adaptation to Life.* Boston: Little, Brown, 1977.

Whelan, Elizabeth. *Preventing Cancer: What You Can Do to Reduce Your Risks Up to 50%.* New York: Norton, 1978.

Williams, Elizabeth Friar. *Notes of a Feminist Therapist.* New York: Praeger, 1976.

Winkler, Win Ann. *Post-Mastectomy.* New York: Hawthorn, 1976.

Woodburn, John C. *Cancer: The Search for Its Origins.* New York: Holt, Rinehart & Winston, 1964.

Some Medical Journals

Breast
CA—A Cancer Journal for Clinicians
Cancer
Cancer Research
Clinical Radiology

International Journal of Cancer
Journal of the American Medical Association
Journal of the National Cancer Institute
Oncology
Radiology
Recent Results in Cancer Research
Yearbook of Cancer

Cumulative Bibliographies

Index Medicus. Extensive bibliography of journal articles in medicine.

Intercom, NCI Breast Cancer Task Force, Cancer Biology and Diagnosis Division, Landow Building, Bethesda, MD 20014. Specialized to breast cancer.

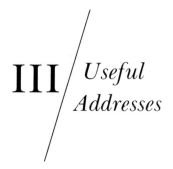

III / Useful Addresses

BEBI (Breast Examination Bras, Inc.), 29 Ainsworth Avenue, East Brunswick, NJ 08816.

Cancer Counseling and Research Center, 1300 Summit Avenue, Suite 710, Fort Worth, TX 76102. Tel. (817) 335-4823.

East West Foundation, 359 Boylston Street, Boston, MA 02116. Tel. (617) 536-3360.

FACT, Ltd. (Foundation for Alternative Cancer Therapies), Box HH, Old Chelsea Station, New York, NY 10011. Tel. (212) 741-2790.

Hippocrates Health Institute, 21 Exeter Street, Boston, MA 02100. Tel. (617) 267-9525.

IACVF (International Association of Cancer Victims and Friends), 434 South San Vincente Boulevard, Los Angeles, CA 90048. Tel. (213) 659-7533. A West Coast information center for nontoxic cancer therapies.

Linus Pauling Institute for Science and Medicine, 2700 Sand Hill Road, Menlo Park, CA 94025.

Make Today Count, P.O. Box 303, 218 South 6th Street, Burlington, IO 52601.

National Health Federation, 212 West Foothill Boulevard, Monrovia, CA 91016. A consumers' health and nutrition action group.

Regenesis, Inc., 18 East 53d Street, New York, NY 10022. Tel. (212) 593-2782. Postmastectomy shop.

S.H.A.R.E. mastectomy/cancer counseling groups, Strang Clinic–Preventive Medicine Institute, 55 East 34th Street, New York, NY 10016.

Index

ABOUT THE AUTHOR

CAROLE SPEARIN MCCAULEY is the author of *Pregnancy After 35; Computers and Creativity; Happenthing in Travel On,* a novel; and *Six Portraits,* a book of computer-assisted fiction. *Surviving Breast Cancer* is her fifth book.

Her background as a science writer includes a stint as medical news reporter at the National Institutes of Health, Bethesda, Maryland. She has worked extensively with feminist groups, including the Woman's Salon, a New York area writers' organization, where she is coordinator of its public events. A versatile writer, her articles, fiction, poetry, satire and interviews have appeared in many magazines, anthologies, and newspapers in the United States and Canada.

She is married and lives in Greenwich, Connecticut.